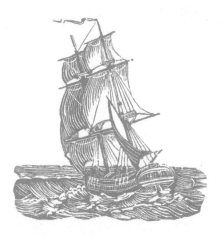

Myth, Fact, *and* Navigators' Secrets

Myth, Fact, *and* Navigators' Secrets

Incredible Tales *of the* Sea and Sailors

J. GREGORY DILL

THE LYONS PRESS
GUILFORD, CONNECTICUT

An imprint of The Globe Pequot Press

The Lyons Press is an imprint of The Globe Pequot Press.

10 9 8 7 6 5 4 3 2 1

Printed in the United States of America

ISBN-10: 1-59228-879-0
ISBN-13: 978-159228-879-3

The Library of Congress Cataloging-in-Publication data is available on file.

To Donna Margaret—

the constant fair wind in my sails

J. G. D.

Contents

Introduction

R eaders should be forewarned that the collection of nautical stories comprising *Myth, Fact, and Navigators' Secrets* is not meant to
be an academic reference source for marine researchers or his-
torians toiling away in dusty stacks of ivy-covered university libraries.

The primary purpose of *Myth, Fact, and Navigators' Secrets* is to entertain—to surprise, amuse, divert, and delight those who love the sea and
enjoy reading about it. If you should learn something while reading, I
apologize.

While *Myth, Fact, and Navigators' Secrets* shamelessly exploits every
ironic instance and every humorous happenstance, it steadfastly refuses
to quash the quirky or conceal the truly tragic in the name of political
correctness.

Some writers create coffee-table books. I conceived *Myth, Fact, and
Navigators' Secrets* as a "head" book (that's bathroom book for you landlubbers!). Stow it in that tiny sanctuary, ready for your reading pleasure
during any visit, long or short. Enjoy!

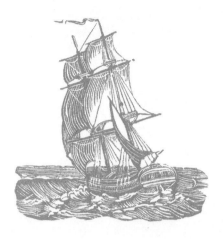

Myth, Fact, *and* Navigators' Secrets

The Recycled Privateer

Early experience as a youthful seaman gave Enos Collins an appreciative eye for the lines of both beautiful women and trim sailing craft. So when his practiced eye fell upon the unusual little vessel on the Halifax waterfront in the fall of 1811, he recognized her as something unique, unlike any other vessel in the harbor—a fast sailer with which a clever man might expect to increase his personal fortune.

A British anti-slaving frigate had arrested *Black Joke*, a classic Baltimore clipper, while she performed the task of ferrying African slaves from a large mother ship to various ports along the Atlantic coast of the southern United States. Now she languished in Halifax Harbor, awaiting her turn at Vice-Admiralty Court where she would be sold by the Crown as confiscated property to someone who would appreciate her particular pecuniary possibilities. Only 54 feet long and with a beam of 18.5 feet, she carried a fore-and-aft schooner rig with square sails on the foremast, as well as three large headsails. Her most striking feature was fore- and mainmasts raked aft at almost twelve degrees, giving her the illusion of speed even as she tugged impatiently at her mooring lines.

Collins, like many a profit-minded New England and Nova Scotian merchant engaged in the sea trade, adhered to the practical philosophy of Ben Franklin, who proclaimed that a man needed only three things in life to be truly happy and prosperous—"an old wife, an old dog, and ready money." Collins may or may not have possessed the first two, but he certainly had plenty of the third. He took £438 of his ready money to purchase *Black Joke* from the Royal Navy Vice-Admiralty Court in November 1811.

Merchants who attended the sale could not imagine Collins using his new craft for legal trade: She was far too small to run profitably as a freighter, and they certainly couldn't see the practical, frugal businessman converting her for use as a personal yacht. But those watching did respect Collins's business savvy and likely expected him to launch *Black Joke* into some kind of illicit activity, possibly into a career of coastal smuggling where her superior speed and maneuverability might be employed to help him avoid paying customs duties to both Uncle Sam and King George. Soon after acquiring the vessel he renamed her *Liverpool Packet*, for his hometown of Liverpool, Nova Scotia.

Political events in 1812, however, overtook Mr. Collins and any plans he may have made for his swift little "trading" vessel. The US Congress, fed up with the Royal Navy's policy of "impressing" American seamen into service in His Majesty's ships, declared war on Great Britain and her colonies and quickly began issuing letters of marque to privately owned and armed privateer vessels to search for, run down, and legally seize British ships at sea (explanations of the terms *letter of marque* and *privateer* appear at the end of this story).

After many frustrating bureaucratic delays, Collins finally managed to secure a British letter of marque from the governor of Nova Scotia, for the purpose of capturing US merchant vessels. The idea of participating in what amounted to legalized piracy appealed to Collins, as he was well aware that he had the perfect instrument for the project in his *Liverpool Packet*. He quickly outfitted the diminutive clipper with the necessary weaponry to chase down American merchant ships, ordering four six-pounder guns and a larger twelve-pounder gun installed on her deck—about the equivalent in firepower today of mounting a 105-millimeter howitzer on a Boston Whaler. *Liverpool Packet's* armament was more than enough to persuade any captain of a slow, lumbering, unarmed Yankee merchantman to come about and surrender.

By October 1812 stable hands, bank clerks, butchers, teachers, and other assorted landlubbers, as well as the marine scum of the waterfronts of Halifax, Liverpool, Boston, and New York, had eagerly signed on an increasing number of British and American privateer vessels. All hoped to make their fortunes by seizing enemy vessels and goods, then sailing them back to home ports to be sold at auction, with the proceeds to be shared among the successful owners, crews, and their respective governments.

When the heavily armed *Liverpool Packet* finally slipped her mooring lines and headed out into the Atlantic, her eager crew under Captain Joseph Barss constantly scanned the horizon by day for any sign of fair game and dreamed in their hammocks at night of running down some fat Boston-bound indiaman carrying a valuable cargo of spices or port wine. In fact, in their wildest dreams, they could never have imagined how successful their hunting would be.

During the remainder of 1812 and into 1813 *Liverpool Packet* sent forty rich prizes back to be sold at Liverpool and Halifax, greatly adding to Collins's personal fortune. But the little Baltimore clipper's luck finally ran out in 1813 when she was overhauled and captured by Captain Shaw of the faster American privateer *Thomas.* Taken to Portsmouth, New Hampshire, *Liverpool Packet* was condemned to be sold by marshal's sale. A group of Boston merchants purchased her, intending to send her out as a licensed US privateer under the name *Young Teazer's Ghost.* (See chapter 41 for the origin of this strange name.) Captain Barss was thrown into the Boston jail for a time before being freed in a prisoner exchange. When Barss finally arrived home in Nova Scotia, his first command was, ironically, *Thomas.* She had, during his incarceration, been captured by the Royal Navy, sailed back to Halifax, and sold at Vice-Admiralty Court.

Young Teazer's Ghost fared badly as a privateer. Disgruntled shareholders looking for more profitable ventures decided to pull their investment by selling her to a group of Portsmouth, New Hampshire, investors who wished to try their luck at privateering. She now bore her third change of name in two years—*Portsmouth Packet.* Unfortunately for this group of investors, *Portsmouth Packet,* while hunting for British merchant shipping in the Bay of Fundy, was surprised and captured off Digby, Nova Scotia, by HMS *Fantom* on October 5, 1813. When *Portsmouth Packet* went through Vice-Admiralty Court again at Halifax, none other than Enos Collins stepped forward at the sale with more of his ready money in hand to purchase the clipper for the second time in two years.

Collins refurbished his vessel, restored her *Liverpool Packet* name, and once again sent her out as a privateer, this time under the command of one Captain Seeley, who managed to bring in only fourteen prizes during 1814. By this time the profit in privateering was becoming lean. Merchant ships on both sides of the conflict now mounted defensive guns and traveled in convoys for protection, making prize capture highly difficult and extremely risky. Collins finally mothballed *Liverpool Packet* and, by the end of the conflict in 1814, decided to invest the war profits generated from his privateering investment in what some might consider another form of legal piracy—founding his own banking firm.

During her privateering life, *Black Joke/Liverpool Packet/Young Teazer's Ghost/Portsmouth Packet* had earned several million dollars, mostly for the sly Enos Collins.

POSTSCRIPT

A *privateer* was a privately owned and armed vessel that, in time of war, cruised against trading vessels of an enemy power with the goal of either destroying or capturing said vessels. The men who crewed privateer vessels were also called privateers. When enemy vessels were captured and returned to a friendly port they were referred to as *prizes*. The owner, captain, and crew of the privateer that made the capture, as well as the state, shared in the proceeds when the enemy ship and her cargo were sold. During the War of 1812 both Britain and the United States made extensive use of privateer vessels to harass the other's sea trade.

A privateer received his authorization for action against enemy ships through a legal document bearing the commission of a sovereign power, known as a *letter of marque*. A letter of marque was worded in such a way as to entirely define the parameters under which the privateer vessel and her crew were to operate, and also served to remind the commission bearer that he was to restrict himself to taking *only* enemy vessels and cargoes, and not drift into the tempting activity of full piracy where any prize might be taken. Examples of both American and British letters of marque follow:

TEXT OF A UNITED STATES LETTER OF MARQUE—WAR OF 1812

JAMES MADISON, President of the United States of America, To All Who Shall See These Presents, Greeting:

Be it Known, That in pursuance of an Act of Congress, passed on the _____ day of _____ one thousand eight hundred and twelve, I have commissioned, and by these presents do commission, the private armed _____ called the _____ of the burthen of ____ tons, or thereabouts, owned by _____ mounting ____ carriage guns, and navigated by _____ men, hereby authorizing _____ Captain and _____ Lieutenant of the said _____ and any other officers and crew thereof, to subdue, seize, and take any armed or unarmed British vessel, public or private, which shall be found within the jurisdictional limits of the United States, or elsewhere on the high seas, or within the waters of the British Dominions, and such captured vessel, with her apparel, guns, and appurtenances, and goods or effects which shall be found on board the same, together with all the British persons and others who shall be found acting on board, to bring within some port of the United States; and also to re-take any vessel, goods, and effects of the people of the United States, which may have been captured by any British armed vessel, in order that the proceedings may be had concerning such capture or recapture in due form of law, and as to right and justice shall appertain.

The said _____ is further authorized to detain, seize, and take all vessels and effects, to whomsoever belonging, which shall be liable thereto according to the law of nations and the rights of the United States as a power at war, and to bring the same within some port of the United States, in order that due proceedings may be had thereupon.

This commission to continue in force during the pleasure of the President of the United States for the time being.

GIVEN under my hand and seal of the United States of America, at the City of Washington, the _____ day of _____ in the year of our Lord, one thousand eight hundred and _____ and of the independence of the said states the _____.

By the President JAMES MADISON
JAMES MONROE Secretary of State

TEXT OF A BRITISH DOMINION LETTER OF MARQUE—WAR OF 1812

Sir **JOHN SHERBROOKE**, Knight of the Most Honourable Order of the Bath, Lieutenant-Governor, and Commander in Chief, in and over His Majesty's Province of Nova Scotia, and its Dependencies, vice Admiral of the same, &c &c

To The Worshipful and Honourable **ALEXANDER CROKE**, L.L.D Judge and Commissionary of His Majesty's Court of Vice Admiralty for the Province &c &c &c

Whereas, by His Majesty's Commission under the Great Seal of Great Britain bearing Date the 13th Day of October in the year of Our Lord 1812, and in the 52d Year of His Majesty's Reign, the Lords Commissioners for executing the Office of Lord High Admiral are required and authorized to issue forth and grant Letters of Marque and Reprisal to any of His Majesty's Subjects or others, whom we shall deem fitly qualified in that Behalf for apprehending, seizing, and taking the Ships, Vessels and Goods belonging to the United States of America, or to any Persons being Subjects of the United States of America (save and except for any Ships to which license has been granted) and to bring the same to Judgement in any of His Majesty's Courts of Admiralty within his Dominions, for Proceedings and Adjudication and Condemnation to be thereupon had, according to the Court of Admiralty, and the Laws of Nations; These are, therefore, to will and require you to cause a Letter of Marque and Reprisals to be issued out of the High Court of Admiralty unto _____ Commander of the _____ Burthern of about ____ Tons, mounted with ___ Carriage Guns carrying Shot of ___ Pounds Weight and navigated with _____ men, whereas the said _____ is commander, to apprehend, seize, and take the Ships, Vessels and Goods Belonging to the United States of America, or to any persons being Subjects of France, according to His Majesty's Commission and Instruction aforesaid. And you are to keep an exact Journal of Proceedings, and therein particularly to take notice of all Prizes taken, the nature of such Prizes, the Time and Place of their being taken, the value of them as near as you can judge, as also the Situation, Motion and Strength of the Americans, as well as you can discover by the best Intelligence you can get; of which you shall from Time to Time as you shall have Opportunity, to transmit an Account to our Secretary. Provide always that security be given according to His Majesty's Instructions before mentioned; the Said Letters of Marque and Reprisal to continue in force until further orders, for which this shall be your Warrant.

Given under my Hand, and the Great Seal of the Province this ____ day of _____ 18 __ in the _____ year of His Majesty's Reign.

By His Excellency's Command.

Fate of the Star of Scotland

November 13, 1942, found the six-masted, 2,290-ton schooner *Star of Scotland* making slow progress nine hundred nautical miles west of the South African coast, on a voyage from Cape Town to the port of Paranagua on the coast of Brazil. Rust stains and corrosion betrayed the advanced age of the steel-hulled vessel as she plodded on laboriously, carrying nothing more valuable than 880 tons of sand ballast. At best, her crew of seventeen mostly inexperienced seamen may have expected to put in just another tedious day like all the others since leaving port—except that the date was Friday the Thirteenth. Likely the old salts among *Star of Scotland's* crew considered the date an unlucky one to be at sea; they may have considered lying low to avoid any kind of "accident" that might befall them during that ill-omened twenty-four-hour period of bad juju.

Those same few of *Star of Scotland's* crew who worried about the unlucky date might also have inclined toward harboring superstitious concerns about the vessel's eclectic history, especially her name and rig changes. Changing a ship's name is still considered by some sailors to be tempting an ill fate. *Star of Scotland* began her sailing career in 1887 as *Kenilworth*, a four-masted bark built for the Waverly Line of Liverpool, England. While at San Francisco in 1889 a fire on board the ship caused heavy damage, which left her a virtual hulk. New owners purchased the damaged vessel, repaired her, and sent her back to sea. In 1908 Alaska Packers' Association of San Francisco bought her and renamed her *Star of Scotland*. Alaska Packers sold her in 1930 to her next owners, who used her as a fishing barge until 1938 when she was again sold, this time to be used as a floating casino under another change of name—*Rex*. In 1941 the East Asiatic Company of Los Angeles bought her, rerigged her as a six-masted schooner, and restored her name—*Star of Scotland*. The US government took over the schooner when America joined World War II after the Japanese attack on Pearl Harbor.

But her past history and changes of name suddenly became moot points when, at five past nine on the morning of November 13, Captain Constantine A. Flink of *Star of Scotland* was startled by the sound of gunfire. Flink quickly discovered that the source of the shooting was the deck gun of a U-boat that had surfaced some distance off. The first shot had passed ahead of the ship without causing damage, but the second and subsequent shells exploded into the tired old schooner's hull. It was obvious to the captain that the U-boat meant to sink his ship. Flink quickly destroyed the ship's signal books and documents, then returned to the deck to discover that the crew had already lowered lifeboats—and in the lowering, the experienced first mate had apparently lost his footing and fallen into the sea. The struggling man soon disappeared from sight as smoke from burning woodwork belowdecks, set alight by the U-boat's gunfire, settled on the water's surface. Flink ran below to the galley to gather up a few provisions. He returned topside with the food, threw it into another lifeboat, then climbed aboard and lowered the lifeboat awkwardly to the water's surface. As he rowed away from the burning, listing schooner, Flink watched the U-boat maneuver toward him before releasing an inflatable boat with armed submariners.

Flink's pursuers easily overtook him, and he was seized and taken aboard the submarine as a prisoner. Kapitanleutnant Helmut Witte of *U-159* interrogated Flink about his ship, cargo, destination, and last port of call. He also explained to the captain that, while he planned to let the schooner's crew go, Flink would have to remain a prisoner aboard the U-boat to prevent him from commanding another enemy ship while the war continued. Flink argued with Witte, telling him in both German and English that most of his crew were inexperienced seamen who did not have the navigational skills to successfully make a landfall without his guidance, as he (Flink) was now the only professional seaman left with experience in navigation. The U-boat commander agreed with Flink that the crew would most likely perish without an experienced man guiding them. Unfortunately, Witte's directives from U-boat command were not negotiable. Orders from headquarters dated just two months before, on September 17, 1942, specifically forbade U-boat commanders from rescuing members of ships sunk, including picking up persons in the water and putting them in lifeboats, righting capsized lifeboats, or providing them with food and water. They were to pick up only captains and chief engineers, who were to be transported to Germany and interned until war's end.

Witte had a very tough decision to make—follow orders and send fifteen men to a likely slow and certain death or give the men at least a sporting chance for survival by allowing their captain to remain with them. For a few moments the German commander weighed his orders against his natural compassion for fellow seamen. Finally he asked Captain Flink if he would be willing to swear not to command another vessel against Germany during the remainder of the war. If Flink agreed, the German would allow the captain to remain with his men. Flink agreed.

Witte's men had by this time captured the crew in the other lifeboat and taken them in tow. Witte gave orders for the submarine to tow the lifeboat about the area to search for the missing first mate, but no trace of the man was found. Witte released Flink to join his men in the lifeboat and ordered his sailors to put additional food and water into the lifeboat for their voyage.

The submarine crew wished the survivors good luck as the lifeboat was released and set adrift. The U-boat submerged, leaving a smoldering *Star of Scotland* sinking lower in the water and Captain Flink and his fifteen crew to fend for themselves. Soon *Star of Scotland* slipped beneath the surface, and the lifeboat was left alone on the sea, save for a patch of floating debris where the schooner had been. Under Flink's instruction, the crew jury-rigged a mast by lashing oars together and made a crude sail from the boat's canvas weather cover. Flink used a small boat compass to set an easterly course to the coast of Africa. The survivors successfully made landfall on the coast of Angola eighteen days later, after a voyage of more than a thousand nautical miles.

During the attack of *U-159* only one of the schooner's crewmen had been lost, not as a direct result of the attack, but because of a shipboard accident—falling overboard while lowering a lifeboat—the kind of mishap that many sailors believe is more likely to happen to an unsuspecting seaman on unlucky Friday the Thirteenth.

Seventeenth-Century Guinness Record?

Quickly now! How many restorationists might you reasonably expect to be able to squeeze into the stern navigational lantern of a naval ship? To answer that very important question we must travel back in time, to the second half of the seventeenth century.

With the restoration of King Charles II to the British throne, the famous diarist, naval reformer, and libertine Samuel Pepys was elevated (through the influence of his patron, the earl of Sandwich) to the rank of clerk of the acts to the Navy Board. This effectively made Pepys one of the most important and powerful officers in England's navy.

Pepys is probably best remembered for the coded diaries in which he recorded events during the Great Fire of London and the horrors of the Black Plague. But few, it seems, know that he was an able and talented administrator responsible for the vigorous modernization of England's then decidedly lackluster navy. His considerable organizational efforts were eventually responsible for building the Royal Navy into the most effective sea force in Europe, resulting in Pepys's eventual rise to the not inconsequential rank of secretary for Admiralty affairs.

But we must look to his struggling early years in the naval service for an answer to the earlier question. During the 1660s Pepys exhibited three main interests—money, sex, and the navy. By wielding his considerable influence, the pursuit of one interest often brought him into contact with the other two. He was constantly sought out by persons wishing to obtain lucrative positions within the naval service, and who were willing to purchase plum placements for themselves or relatives. Frequently this involved Pepys happily receiving plain brown envelopes containing cash or, less frequently, the offer of the "favors" of the daughter or wife of a man seeking a dockyard position—the trysts taking place in Pepys's Admiralty offices.

Pepys's position also required that he frequently entertain the wives of his patron, Lord Sandwich, and other noble acquaintances, a chore that Pepys's libidinous nature no doubt relished. One afternoon in the winter of 1661 Pepys found himself engaged in amusing a group of high-born ladies and their servants by conducting them on a tour of the hundred-gun HMS *Royal Sovereign*. At a time when a fighting ship's power was often judged by the size of her main stern lantern, *Royal Sovereign* had just about the biggest one around. And in a lark worthy of inclusion in the *Guinness Book of World Records*, had it then existed, Pepys convinced the female companions he was guiding that they should try to discover how many of their number might fit inside the enormous navigational lantern mounted on the vessel's stern. His diary entry for January 17, 1661, reads in part:

> . . . my Lady Sandwich, my Lady Jemimah, Mrs. Brown, Mrs. Grace, and Mary and the page, my lady's servants, and myself went into the Lanthorne together . . . [*lanthorne*, of course, was the seventeenth century term for "lantern"].

So if anyone should ask you, *seven* restorationists can intimately squeeze into a ship's lantern. Or perhaps it would be more correct to say six, and one lecherous, financially secure naval bureaucrat.

The Accidental Steamboat Race

enry Burden was a Scottish immigrant and master ironmonger who left his homeland in 1819 to seek his fortune in America. The newly arrived Scot had little trouble finding a job with agricultural implement maker Townsend and Corning of Albany because of his special skills in fabricating iron products. In no time he was producing vastly improved farming implements and machines for the company, including the first successful mechanical cultivator designed in the United States. By 1822 Burden had acquired controlling interest in the failing Troy Iron and Nail factory, quickly turning that operation into one of the largest and most profitable iron foundries in the country. His genius and financial expertise allowed him to accumulate the wealth that would permit him to cultivate yet another interest he keenly wished to pursue.

Burden turned his fertile imagination to a subject that had intrigued him since first arriving in America—river navigation using steam power. It had been almost twenty-six years since residents along the Hudson River had witnessed Robert Fulton's steamboat *Clermont* wheezing across the waters, and there had been little in the way of innovation in steamboat design since *Clermont*'s success. A quarter century later steamboats were still being fitted with poorly designed and badly crafted boilers that blew up with such astounding regularity, travelers felt compelled to set their estates in order before booking passage.

Burden knew he could design and build a better steam-powered vessel—one that would be safer, faster, and more economical than anything then thrashing about on the river. In 1833 he began construction of a passenger and freight steam vessel of a radically different design from anything then plying the Hudson. He named his new boat *Helen*, in honor of his wife. *Helen* (the boat, not the wife) incorporated a single 24-foot-diameter paddle wheel that operated between twin pontoon-like hulls more than 150 feet in length. The paddle wheel was driven by a single-cylinder steam engine having a piston twenty-four inches in diameter—the engine and boiler being of Burden's own design and construction.

Placing the wheel inboard (between) the pontoons vastly improved the efficiency of the wheel's action on the water, which meant the engine could be smaller and thus use less fuel per mile traveled. Using his unique double-hull design meant that Burden's boat would draw less water than similar-sized craft and would ensure that *Helen* could navigate the shallower waters of the river. The first tests with *Helen* revealed she could easily achieve a speed of fifteen miles per hour, with her single large wheel making seven revolutions per minute to attain that speed. That feat was achieved using an engine needing to generate only 25 percent of the power required to drive a similar-sized conventional vessel— a fact that would have warmed the hearts of any early environmentalists living along the shores of the Hudson.

The successful initial testing of his completed boat suggested to Burden that *Helen*'s speed might be increased to twenty miles per hour. To that end Burden invited a few of his friends (those who would be most likely to invest in his idea and who had the stomach for the danger involved) to depart for a day's cruising on the Hudson River. At 7 AM on July 14, 1833, *Helen* slipped away from the dock some twenty minutes after the departure of the then fastest steamer on the river, *Erie*. Burden had evidently planned to turn this outing into a full-fledged steamboat race by choosing to leave after *Erie*, then overtaking her in a dramatic show of *Helen*'s superior speed. *Erie* was then about six miles ahead of *Helen*, belching great sooty clouds of smoke and leaving a substantial area of disturbed water in her wake because of her inefficient hull and paddle-wheel design. In contrast *Helen* seemed to glide upon the water, hardly disturbing the surface at all because of her streamlined, pointed hulls—moving forward like a graceful swan following in the turbulent wake of a blundering hippopotamus. As it became obvious to bystanders along the river that the two boats intended to race, crowds began forming along both shores to witness the spectacle and bet on the outcome.

Fifty minutes after leaving the dock, *Helen* easily overtook a small steamboat, *Champion*, traveling in the same direction near Dobbs Ferry. *Helen*'s paddle wheel was now turning at nearly eighteen revolutions per minute, with still more throttle available to Burden. By the time *Helen* neared Poughkeepsie at 12:20 PM, she was fairly flying across the water at twenty miles per hour, and she had reduced the distance between herself and *Erie* by half, or three miles. This was all the more remarkable because, unknown to Burden, the crew of *Erie* had anticipated a race with *Helen* and decided to improve their chances by cheating. They had stowed aboard their boat large quantities of tar and turpentine to throw on the fuel to induce higher burn temperatures in their boiler's fireboxes and thereby produce more steam and greater speed.

Fate, however, was to intervene. Just as Burden's boat was about to triumphantly overtake *Erie*, a cutoff valve gear failed, causing *Helen*'s speed to immediately fall off. Disheartened, Burden ordered the engine stopped so temporary repairs could be made. It was almost 3 PM by the time *Helen* finally got under way again, with *Erie* by then well out of sight. But more technical problems ensued for Burden's boat, including boiler leaks that prevented *Helen* from regaining her impressive early speeds.

Helen's unfortunate failure in the unofficial race with *Erie* didn't dim Burden's enthusiasm for his marine designs, though. And despite her initial public failure, newspaper accounts of the race and of *Helen*'s unusual design features, efficiency, and speed soon spread. When the news reached Britain, an English naval spy was dispatched to have a peek at Burden's boat. But the English agent never got a chance to see the radically new craft perform. Shortly after her racing disappointment against *Erie*, *Helen* had some additional bad luck; some said damned bad luck, for she was reduced to a total wreck after accidentally running squarely into the Castleton dam. Burden, however, survived and went on to patent many of his innovative marine designs. He eventually succeeded in constructing an even bigger and better boat four years after the loss of *Helen*.

Invitation to a Duel at Sea

The strange tale of the duel between two equally matched fighting ships, the US Frigate *Chesapeake* and His Britannic Majesty's Frigate *Shannon*, and the two men who commanded them, has almost been forgotten.

In 1813 America's second war with Britain was almost a year old. The young US Navy had humbled Britain's mighty war fleet in a number of humiliating defeats at sea, giving the USN a much-needed morale boost.

Chesapeake was just completing a refit when Captain James Lawrence (thirty-two and fresh from a well-publicized victory over HMS *Peacock* while he was in command of USS *Hornet*) arrived at Boston to take up his new command. Lawrence was a man of immense personal ambition, and tales of his brilliant sea victory over *Peacock* had become the stuff of legend among seamen of both the Royal Navy and the USN. Although ambitious, Lawrence genuinely wished to free his country's shores of King George's menacing ships and end the detestable practice by the British of boarding American merchant vessels and forcibly impressing American citizens into Royal Navy service.

Chesapeake and Lawrence would soon find an able adversary in the form of *Shannon* and her captain, Phillip de Vere Broke, a veteran of the wars with Napoleon's Republican Navy and a man who was in the habit of constantly drilling his men at small arms, boarding, and exercising *Shannon*'s "great guns." Broke's ambition was to secure advancement for himself within the Royal Navy through a successful engagement with any American fighting ship. Such a victory would also help Britain regain lost international prestige for her once great Royal Navy. Lawrence and Broke were cut from the same cloth—both brave and fiercely loyal to their respective heads of state. Had the two men met in peacetime, they might have expected to become good friends.

Lawrence arrived at his new command to find *Chesapeake* a troubled and undermanned ship. Her previous captain (Evans) had been a weak and ineffective commander. *Chesapeake*'s senior officers were all ill or reposted, and the crew was unhappy that prize money owed them from previous sea actions had still not been paid. Lawrence was dismayed to find that his first lieutenant was only twenty-one years old and had little experience in battle. The remaining lieutenants were all just boys in their teens, and only recently had been midshipmen. To add to Lawrence's problems, the merchants of Boston began to pressure him to drive the British menace from their coast. They were unaware, however, that his orders specifically forbade him to engage armed enemy ships. He was instead ordered to proceed north with *Chesapeake* to the Gulf of St. Lawrence, where he was to harass and capture unarmed enemy merchant vessels convoying between Britain and Quebec.

Meanwhile Broke's dirty little *Shannon*, badly in need of provisions and a refit, tacked repeatedly across the entrance to Boston Harbor, brazenly tempting *Chesapeake* to come out and fight. Captain Broke took the taunting one step further by actually sending a series of letters to Captain Lawrence (via Boston fishermen) inviting him to a ship duel at some prearranged point off the coast. One letter began: "Sir, I request you will do me the favor to meet the *Shannon* with her [*Chesapeake*], ship to ship, to try the fortune of our respective flags." Incredibly, Broke went on to describe the number and size of *Shannon*'s guns and the number of her crew, and ended the letter with ". . . favor me with a speedy reply. We are short of provisions and water and cannot stay long here."

Indeed, morale aboard *Shannon* was falling as fresh water and food rations began to run low. The crew was tired and bored with the waiting game and itching for a little shore time at *Shannon*'s base in Halifax, Nova Scotia.

Finally on June 1, *Chesapeake*'s refit was completed. Lawrence forbade his first officer to mention the existence of Broke's letters to anyone, lest the secretary of the navy gain wind of them. *Chesapeake* made sail at noon, heading out of Boston Harbor in search of *Shannon*. Following in *Chesapeake*'s wake was a flotilla of fishing craft and yachts crammed with picnic lunches, liquor, and eager Boston citizens in a holiday mood, expecting to witness a quick and decisive victory for the celebrated naval hero Lawrence. *Chesapeake* found *Shannon* twenty nautical miles from the harbor mouth, and the two ships immediately cleared for action and began maneuvering for favorable winds.

When the distance between the two vessels closed to two miles, some of *Chesapeake*'s crew refused to man their guns without some assurance that they would get the prize money owed them from previous enemy engagements under Captain Evans. With only minutes left before the opening shots, Lawrence ordered his purser to issue chits for prize payments to the few mutinous crewmen.

Slowly the vessels closed to the range of a pistol shot. At 5:50 PM the first broadsides were exchanged, wreaking great damage upon both vessels. Lawrence was wounded in the first minutes of action, but remained on deck giving commands as the two vessels inadvertently collided, each becoming entangled in the other's rigging. Broke saw this as an advantage and ordered "boarders away" to *Chesapeake*'s main deck. Broke was almost immediately grazed but unhurt by a musket ball fired by a marine sharpshooter high up in *Chesapeake*'s maintop. As the smoke of battle settled upon the decks of *Chesapeake*, Lawrence received another more serious wound and was then taken below to the surgeon.

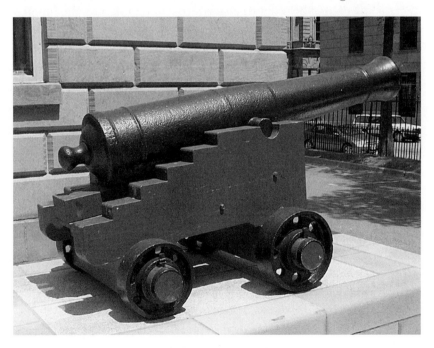

This gun, peacefully guarding the Nova Scotia legislature today, took part in the bloody action aboard HMS Shannon *when she engaged the US Frigate* Chesapeake *off Boston Light on June 1, 1813.* ©2005 by J. Gregory Dill

While bloody hand-to-hand fighting raged on deck above him, *Chesapeake*'s captain uttered those immortal words that have since become part of US Navy tradition—"Don't give up the ship!" Captain Lawrence then lapsed into unconsciousness.

Shannon finally won victory, but not before Captain Broke had suffered a severe cutlass wound to his head. Both Lawrence and Broke were hovering near death from their wounds, unaware of the engagement's outcome. *Chesapeake*'s crew were rounded up and manacled, then locked belowdecks in their own ship. The yachts and fishing boats lying off from the action began returning to Boston, their passengers unsure of the final outcome of the battle because smoke and fog had obscured much of the action. Most believed *Chesapeake* was pursuing *Shannon* out to sea.

When *Shannon* and her prize finally gained Halifax Harbor, news of the capture of an American frigate quickly traveled throughout the town, and the citizens assumed a festive mood. But when the public learned that *Chesapeake*'s captain was the famous James Lawrence, and that he had died of his wounds just before entering harbor, the mood of celebration diminished significantly. Lawrence had assumed the status of a folk hero, even among his British enemies. The respectful light in which the British held Lawrence demanded that the American captain be accorded the full honors of a Royal Navy funeral, one befitting a valiant foe. Even the British army had a part to play. Halifax garrison orders for June 7, 1813, read:

A Funeral Party will be furnished to-morrow, by the 64th Regiment consisting of 300 Rank and File, with a proper proportion of Officers, and to be supplied with three rounds of blank cartridges each man; to inter the Remains of Captain Lawrence, late of the American frigate Chesapeake from the King's Wharf, at half past one o'clock p.m.

The Band of that Corps will attend, and the Party will be commanded by Lieut. Col. Sir J. Wardlow.

The Officers and Garrison will be pleased to attend the Commandant there, at a quarter before two, to march in procession wearing a piece of black crape round their left arm.

(signed) F. T. Thomas,
Major of Brigade

Lawrence's coffin, draped with the American flag, was borne through the streets of Halifax on a carriage accompanied by senior captains of the Halifax Station, while minute guns were fired from the city's citadel fortress—a fitting tribute, and a much better end for Lawrence than a certain court-martial back in Boston, had he lived.

Captain Broke did recover from his wounds after many months, but was never the same. Deeply religious, he lived out his final years guilt-ridden, having learned that he had personally killed (albeit in self-defense) *Chesapeake*'s acting chaplain during hand-to-hand fighting on *Chesapeake*'s main deck.

Chesapeake was repaired and commissioned into the Royal Navy, becoming HMS *Chesapeake*. When she was finally broken up in England years later, timber from her gun deck was sold and used in constructing a gristmill. *Chesapeake Mill* still stands today on the River Meon at the village of Whickham in Hampshire, a testament to that battle between the frigates *Chesapeake* and *Shannon*, a bloody sea duel that, in the final analysis, had little or no strategic significance.

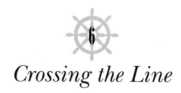

Crossing the Line

The origin of the celebrated "crossing the line" ceremony—the initiation of sailors crossing the equator for the first time—has never been fully documented.

Ancient sailors were a superstitious lot, to say the least. They appreciated how unnatural it was for man to move upon great waters, and so made obsequious pleas to the ruler of the seas, Neptunus Rex (and his earlier incarnation, Poseidon), in the hope that this deity might be cajoled into keeping wind and wave within tolerable limits and compel whatever sea monsters might dwell in his watery domain to refrain from lunching upon poor seamen and their frail craft.

Earliest rites would have been performed upon completion of a safe passage around a prominent promontory, or when beginning to sail down the latitudes of ancient Mediterranean ports. One documented ceremony, conducted by King Hanno of Carthage upon his fleet's safe passage through the Pillars of Hercules (Straits of Gibraltar) in the sixth century BCE, involved the king constructing a coastal shrine to honor Poseidon for his invaluable assistance.

We can probably blame the Vikings for introducing a second element into the present crossing-the-line ceremony—hazing. Hazing of untried hands during passage south across certain parallels might include dunking or dragging a novice sailor for a distance in frigid waters as a test of his endurance and resolve. If the soggy, salt-stained supplicant successfully survived, he was deemed satisfactory to join the seasoned crew. When Viking raiders later began colonizing the shores of Britain, Ireland, and France, they brought their hazing rituals with them. In time, versions of saltwater dunking joined already well-established Roman-based "thank gods we made it!" traditions.

A remnant of the old Viking hazing rite appears in this passage from Captain Woodes Rodgers's log for September 25, 1708:

This day, according to custom, we duck'd those that had never pass'd the Tropick [of Cancer] before. The manner of doing it was by a Rope thro a block from the Main-Yard, to hoist 'em above half way up the Yard, and let 'em fall at once into the Water, having a Stick cross thro their Legs, and well fastened to the Rope, that they might not be surpriz'd and let go their hold. This prov'd of great use to our fresh-water Sailors, to recover the Colour of their Skins, which were grown black and nasty.

Seventeenth-century French sailors may have been first to experience a combined version of Viking and Roman elements. Typically the second mate would appear on deck dressed as Neptune, carrying a large, ornately carved wooden sword with which he would proceed to savagely beat the initiate. A Viking-like "blessing" followed in the form of a bucket of refreshing cold seawater thrown on the bruised and possibly unconscious novice.

Today celebrations of a contemporary sailor's first crossing of the equator will likely include Neptune appearing on deck in kingly attire. His wife, Queen Amphitrite (possibly a hairy bosun in drag), and a retinue that may include the royal baby, a barber, and other assorted assistants embarrass and playfully harass the novices, who are called "pollywogs." After the initiates are good-naturedly tormented for a time by Neptune and his retinue, they are presented to his royal personage, then are either dunked in a barrel of water or tossed into the ship's swimming pool. The ceremony usually ends with the presentation of a parchment document certifying that the holder has officially graduated from pollywog status to become a "shellback" and has undergone official initiation into the "mysteries of the sea."

In the end this much-evolved rite of crossing the line also serves as a bond between contemporary sailors and all those venerable seamen whose vessels plowed ancient, uncharted seas.

Dictionary Gave Sailors a Bad Rap

Nathaniel Bailey was a lexicographer who published a two-volume dictionary in 1737 (George Washington was only five years old at the time, and the future King George III was but a twinkle in his mother's eye). Bailey's *An Universal Etymological English Dictionary* contains what can only be interpreted as a decidedly biased view of the many seamen of the period who could find no employment on seagoing vessels because of depressed economic conditions. Thousands of these men began begging in the streets of London and other English ports.

In Bailey's dictionary, under the subtitle *A collection of the Canting Words and Terms, both ancient and modern, used by Beggars, Gypsies, Cheats, House-Breakers, Shop-Lifters, Foot-Pads, Highway-Men, &c.,* Bailey gives a sampling of what he calls "tar terms" that had entered the slang of the streets through those unfortunate, unemployed seamen.

Not only is this addition to the dictionary interesting from a sociological perspective (with so much poverty and hunger, it is not surprising that hundreds of different words were developed to describe thieves, prostitutes, and con artists), but a number of the terms defined were distinctly nautical in nature, or associated with life at sea. With the government unable or unwilling to assist the welfare of "wasted" seamen, many old salts were reduced to begging and thieving to survive. Bailey evidently felt it safer to assume all begging seamen were criminals who should be dealt with harshly. Following is a sample of the nautical terms and definitions in the dictionary, in Bailey's own words, and associated with his personal view of "criminal" seaman:

Ark-Ruffians—Rogues, who in Conjunction with Watermen & c. rob and sometimes murder on the Water, by picking a Quarrel with the Passenger and then plundering and murdering, stripping and throwing him or her over board.

Barnacles—the Irons worn in Gaol by Felons

Bowse—Drink, or to drink

Captain-Hackham—a fighting, blustering Bully

to Dock—to lie with a Woman

Ebb Tide—when there is little Money in the Pocket

Fire-Ship—a poxed Whore

Half Seas over—almost drunk

Hen-peckt-Frigate—whose Commander and Officers are absolutely swayed by their Wives.

Humpty-Dumpty—Ale boiled with Brandy [a favorite tar tot of
the period]

Land-Lubbers—Vagabonds that beg and steal about the county

Light-Frigate—a young Whore; also a Cruiser

Mumper—a sort of genteel beggar, reckoned the 47th order of
canter or gipsies, who will not accept victuals, but of money or
clothes.

The Male Mumper—sometimes he will appear like a decay'd
gentleman who has been ruined by the South-Sea Scheme [the
South Sea Bubble of 1720, a financial hoax that ruined thousands of marine investors and caused the loss of employment
for thousands of British seaman] or some other unforeseen
folly.

Painter—I'll cut your Painter for ye; I'll prevent your doing me
any Mischief: the Tar Cant when they quarrel with each other.

[A painter is a line attached to the bow of a small boat and used for towing or securing it to a dock.]

Plate Fleet comes in—when money comes to Hand [possibly the origin of the saying *when my ship comes in*]

Rufflers—notorious Rogues who, under Pretence of being maimed Seamen, implore the charity of well disposed Persons, and fail not to watch Opportunities either to steal, break open Houses, or even commit Murder.

Shot Betwixt Wind and Water—Clapt or Pox'd

Spanish-Money—fair words and Compliments

Tackle—a Mistress

Whip Jacks—counterfeit Mariners begging with false Passes, pretending Ship-wrecks, great Losses at Sea, narrow Escapes, & c., telling dismal stories, having learnt Tar Terms on purpose; but are meer cheats; and will not stick to rob a Booth at a Fair, or an House in some By-road. They often carry their Morts or Wenches with them, which they pretend to be their Wives, whom they miraculously saved in the Shipwreck, altho' all their children were drowned, the Ship splitting on a Rock near Lands-End, with such forgeries.

Unfortunately Bailey's dictionary may be responsible for initiating nearly three centuries of character-bashing for sailors, who are still often viewed as unsavory persons, not to be fully trusted. Some of these ideas had also been perpetuated by Dr. Samuel Johnson, who later used Bailey's work as the basis of his own famous English dictionary.

Risky Proposition for Propositioning Women

E ngland in 1670 was probably not the safest place for fashion-conscious women seeking sailor-husbands, as suggested by the wording of an act of Parliament regarding the use of "devices for the contrivance of beauty."

The act was directed at women

... of whatever age, rank, profession, or degree; whether virgin maids or widows; that shall after the passing of this act, impose upon and betray into matrimony any of His Majesty's male subjects, by scents, paints, cosmetics, washes, artificial teeth, false hair, Spanish wool, iron stays, hoops, high-heeled shoes, or bolstered hips, shall incur the penalty of the laws now in force against witchcraft, sorcery, and such like misdemeanours, and that the marriage, upon conviction, shall stand null and void.

Evidently this act was an attempt to aid the navy in keeping men aboard their ships and out of the clutches of women who would keep their men ashore.

The American Coast Pilot *of 1817*

P ilot books, those dry but necessary navigational books found aboard all oceangoing ships to this day, are probably not what the average off-watch sailor would choose to read for entertainment. But finding a pilot book that is almost two hundred years old can prove irresistible for anyone with a sincere interest in nautical history.

The publication of the first *American Coast Pilot* in 1796 established Edmund M. Blunt as a respected author and publisher of accurate

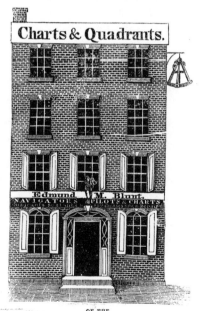

Blunt's ad for his New York marine store.
Courtesy J. Gregory Dill (from his collection)

coastal navigation data for seamen. Blunt was also the publisher who coaxed and cajoled an obscure hardware store clerk named Nathaniel Bowditch to author the now legendary *New American Practical Navigator*, published by Blunt in 1802.

The author's ninth-edition copy of Edmund M. Blunt's popular *American Coast Pilot* was published in New York in 1817 and was owned at some point by a sailor named James Balls of Norfolk, Virginia, if one can believe the name stamped and signed in a flowing hand on the title page. Mr. Balls would have found his *Pilot* absolutely indispensable for sailing directions, whether voyaging to Port Royal, Jamaica, or the fishing grounds of Georges Bank.

A bit of advertising supporting the usefulness of the *Pilot* for seamen appears in the first few pages of Blunt's book with a news story quoted from the *Newburyport Herald* of June 21, 1808:

A sloop belonging to Dartmouth, from Kennebeck, with lumber, in the violent blow of Saturday, upset 16 leagues from our bar, her deck load was washed off, when she righted, and came in by the assistance of Blunt's *Coast Pilot* . . .

The *Pilot* confidently offered seamen advice (for the most part still surprisingly accurate) regarding courses and distances, locations of navigational lights and marker buoys, as well as soundings (depth of water) and shoal hazards from the Gulf of Mexico to as far north as the Gulf of St. Lawrence and Labrador. Even a detailed account of the position, rate of flow, and temperature of the Gulf Stream (much of the data culled by Blunt from the investigations and writings of Benjamin Franklin) was included.

Blunt felt compelled to warn those heading to the Caribbean about navigational treachery practiced by some local seamen. He urged that navigators:

. . . be cautious, while crossing the Bahama Bank, never to follow vessels, if they alter their course often; as the New-Providence Wreckers have frequently decoyed them for the purpose of plunder . . . This is not published to give offence to anyone, but it applies to some of the Providence Navigators, and it is our duty to point out danger to Mariners, from which the Editor will never deviate, or hide from investigation.

In the matter of marine law of the time, Blunt advised the mariner to become thoroughly acquainted with various legislative acts, including the following:

The Legislature of Nova Scotia have enacted that any person convicted of stealing from any vessel wrecked on the coast of that province or the Isle of Sable . . . . shall suffer death.

Blunt also quoted from US federal marine law directing the quantity and kinds of food and water required to be carried by every US-flagged vessel bound across the Atlantic. Depending upon the number of passengers and crew each ship carried, captains were instructed to have the following "well secured under deck":

. . . at least sixty gallons of water, one hundred pounds of salted fresh meat, and one hundred pounds of wholesome ship bread, for every person on board . . . [These victuals would be over and above any live chickens, pickled herring, or pigs brought aboard by passengers wishing to dine on more tasty fare.]

In the matter of the shipping act as it applied to the slave trade, Blunt advised ships' masters:

Any person who imports or causes to be imported into the territory of Louisiana a slave from without the limits of the United States, forfeits for each slave $300, and such slave shall be entitled to, and receive his or her freedom.

When discussing navigating to Newburyport, Blunt noted that the local Marine Society, in the interest of securing sailors' safety, had ". . . built a number of huts and stocked them with fireworks, fuel, straw and food for the use of any castaways thrown upon Plum Island." But he quickly went on to lament the destruction of those huts due to what he described as "the wantonness of individuals and companies, who frequent this spot in the warm season, on parties of pleasure."

One interesting insight into Blunt's character is revealed by a notation on page 211 of the *Pilot* concerning his dealings with a businessman in New Orleans. Evidently Blunt and a Mr. Touro had had a difference of opinion about moneys owed for marine goods and services. Blunt decided to devote a whole page of his *Pilot* to the dispute, giving minute details of the financial arrangement with Touro, and ending with the terse statement:

> Why, Mr. Touro, protest a draft for non-acceptance, when, after paying it, you admit a balance due me of 648 dollars? You shall have the whole truth.

Blunt ended his tirade with the damning words: "Character often survives life!"

It was Edmund Blunt's energy and talent, more than any other American marine publisher of the early nineteenth century, that contributed to the rapid and safe expansion of America's sea power and trade. Americans should know his name as well as that of famed navigational specialist Nathaniel Bowditch.

10

She *and* Her *No Longer Nautical Terms*

L*loyd's List,* that perennial purveyor of no-nonsense nautical news since 1734, shocked its readership a few years ago by announcing the adoption of a new and controversial editorial policy—any ship mentioned in its pages henceforth would be referred to as *it* rather than the traditional feminine forms *she* or *her.*

List editor Julian Bray, apparently unconcerned with causing consternation in the cockpit and bewilderment on the bridge, said he wanted to bring the publication into line with editorial policies current with other business news organizations. Bray told the *Financial Times*:

> Ultimately they [ships] are commodities . . . not things that have characters . . .

The ancient association of the female gender with ships extends back perhaps thousands of years, having evolved from sailors' comparison of the idiosyncrasies of seagoing vessels to those they felt they perceived in the women in their lives. Sailors saw their ships as animate objects needing regular, careful attention, and to which they trusted and devoted their working lives. Plautus, a Greek writing in the second century BCE, and evidently of a sexist bent, noted:

> If a man be seeking trouble he need only buy a ship or take a wife; both will always need trimming.

Almost a millennium later the *Universal Etymological English Dictionary* offered a comparison of a frigate *well rigged* to *a Woman, well drest and genteel.*

The last fifty years have seen life at sea change dramatically. Women have proven their capabilities by making grueling single-handed circumnavigations and have taken their rightful place on the bridges of the world's navies and merchant marines, where skill and expertise are the most important factors and the captain's sex inconsequential. But the fondness with which most sailors refer to their ships in the feminine gender will probably not disappear anytime soon, regardless of the editorial policies of Mr. Bray's *List.*

What other nautical language changes might the *List* be considering for the future? Perhaps we might soon expect to read in the famous publication something as absurd as the following:

> . . . at the time of the impact the ship was proceeding on cruise control with no one in its driver's seat. The captain was in the bathroom and the first mate had gone downstairs to the kitchen for a double latte. Nearly ten minutes had transpired before the Coast Guard finally received the radio call—help! help! help!

Dining at Sea, In Style (1796)

Refrigeration, alcohol and gas stoves, and TV chef Martin Yan have all helped free sailors from the dietary drudgery once common at sea. About the biggest mealtime dilemma well-equipped cruisers have now is deciding whether to crack open a bottle of Chianti from the hills of Sienna or one of those brave New World reds from Chile to accompany that succulent sirloin sizzling back aft on the barbie. Even tomato-juice-sipping vegetarian voyagers can choose to munch on freshly thawed dandelion greens or cauliflower should they so desire, even when sailing in mid-Pacific.

But the choice of food available to our late-eighteenth-century seafaring forefathers was distinctly more modest, as evidenced by the following list of daily rations to be issued to Royal Navy tars of 1796:

> Every man to be allowed daily provisions, as follows, vis
>
> Sunday. One pound of biscuit, one gallon of small beer, one pound of pork, and a half-a-pint of Pease.
>
> Monday. One pound of biscuit, one gallon of small beer, one pint of oatmeal, two ounces of butter, and four ounces of cheese.
>
> Tuesday. One pound of biscuit, one gallon of small beer, and two pounds of beef.
>
> Wednesday. One pound of biscuit, one gallon of small beer, half-a-pint of Pease, a pint of oatmeal, two ounces of butter, four ounces of cheese. [Small beer, by the way, is watered-down beer.]

The remainder of the week was simply a dreary repetition of the same. After some time at sea, however, the crew could expect an additional bit of protein in the form of weevils, which eventually would burrow into all stored foodstuffs. No doubt the generous daily ration of

160 ounces of beer helped the crew overlook the little critters scurrying about at the bottom of their food bowls.

Adding to crews' dreary dietary dilemma was the fact that naval vessels' chefs de cuisine rarely had the benefit of formal culinary training. The main prerequisite for the position of cook seems to have been that the applicant had made some significant anatomical sacrifice—an eye, leg, or arm—while in the service of His Britannic Majesty's Navy. In any British naval vessel after the Battle of Trafalgar, it was difficult to find a cook who still had all of the appendages with which he had been born. Many a tattered man-of-war vet welcomed assignment to the less arduous duty as ship's cook.

One of the cook's duties required that he maintain a large wooden "steep tub" where chunks of pickled pork and beef were soaked to remove the salt used in preserving. The meat was stirred about with a large wooden ladle, or the cook's wooden leg, and was ready for consumption by the lusty carnivores aboard when it floated to the oily surface of the tub. In a rough sea the chef de cuisine would often be kept busy retrieving pieces of salted meat that had escaped over the side of the tub, leaving greasy trails as they slithered about the pitching deck.

Foreign voyages did, however, hold some promise of dietary relief from the monotonous daily provisions. At such times, and depending on the next port of call on the ship's voyage, the crew might look forward to fresh tropical fruit, raisins, currants, olive oil, mutton, pickled beef suet, and the substitution of brandy, rum, or arrack (made from fermented coconut palm sap) in place of the beer allowance. But this additional simple food could never hope to approach the variety of fare available to latter-day mariner-gastronomes.

Nautical Book Tells Two Stories

A nyone who enjoys collecting marine books may recall the thrill of making a truly interesting discovery in some out-of-the-way used-book store. Such was the case one day when I reached for a book that had obviously seen severe service. I carefully examined the gold-embossed cover sporting the title *A New Method of Finding a Ship's Position at Sea* by Captain Thomas H. Sumner. A quick examination of the title page told me it was the third edition of the book, dated 1851. A momentary twitch of disappointment probably crossed my face before I

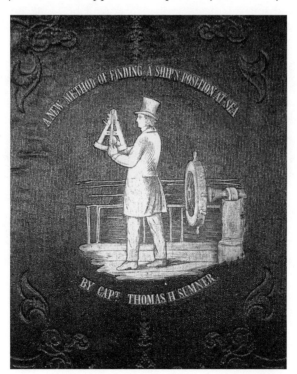

Cover artwork of the author's copy of Sumner's 1851 edition.
©2005 by J. Gregory Dill

reasoned that even a third edition had value, especially because Captain Sumner's first edition of 1837 had so completely revolutionized the practice of navigation at sea.

I put on my best poker face to confront the owner of the shop for a price, lest she see just how badly I wanted that musty, dusty little volume. I counted myself lucky when I paid the few dollars the owner requested. Granted, the book did have some water damage, as evidenced by the warping of the cover, but that only served to prove its long service as a once valued nautical reference of some "hands-on" nineteenth-century navigator.

Sometimes, however, old books have more than one tale to tell, and this book would turn out to be one of them. Examining the book after arriving home, I discovered at the top of the first page, written in a bold and flowing hand, the name *W. H. Gladding*—no doubt the owner's name, I thought. Below the name were the letters *USRS*, which I later learned stood for "United States Revenue Service." There were also scribbled position calculations on every available square inch of the

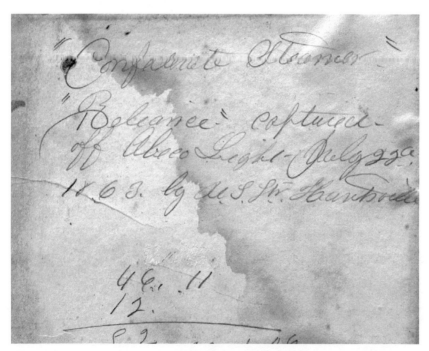

The abbreviated note recording the capture of Gladding's Reliance.
©2005 by J. Gregory Dill

page. On the inside front cover, facing the first page, I eventually noticed a tantalizing notation in a different hand. It read:

Confederate Steamer *Reliance* captured off Abaco Light July 22, 1862 by USS *Huntsville.*

Intrigued by the inscriptions, I became determined to find out what I could about Mr. Gladding, *Reliance,* and *Huntsville.* After a few days of research, I had some answers. *Huntsville,* it turned out, was a single-screw, 840-ton steamer launched in New York in 1857 as a commercial vessel. She was chartered by the US Navy in 1861 and later purchased by the navy for Civil War service as USS *Huntsville,* after undergoing conversion to a gunboat. It was while she was serving on patrol duty in the Bahama Channel and the Gulf of Mexico, enforcing the blockade of Confederate coastal waters and under command of Acting Volunteer Lieutenant William C. Rogers, that she had chased down Gladding's *Reliance.* The following is the text of Lieutenant Rogers's report to Secretary of the Navy Gideon Welles regarding the capture of the Confederate steamer *Reliance* and Lieutenant Gladding:

USS *Huntsville,* Bahama Channel, July 21, 1862
SIR:
I have the honor to report to you the capture this day of the rebel steamer *Reliance,* three days out from Doboy Bar, Ga., bound to Nassau with a cargo of 243 bales sea-island cotton.

I fell in with her soon after daylight, a little to eastward of Abaco, and after a chase of about 30 miles, succeeded in bringing her to, after firing 14 shot and shell.

She is commanded by Lieutenant Gladding, formerly of the Navy and revenue service, and since the rebellion in command of the schooner *Parliament,* in which he has several times run the blockade.

The *Reliance* was chased on leaving Doboy by one of the blockading fleet, but escaped by superior speed.

I regret extremely not being able to either send or tow this prize to Boston, agreeably to your circular, but she had fuel for only six hours, and my own coal was very nearly exhausted, and would but take us to Key West, to which port I am now towing her.

Please find enclosed list of officers and muster roll of crew of the *Huntsville.*

Respectfully, your obedient servant,
WM. C. ROGERS,
Acting Volunteer Lieutenant, Commanding.

Hon. GIDEON WELLES,
Secretary of the Navy, Washington, D.C.

It is curious that there is a day difference between the book notation and Rogers's report to Secretary Welles. But the following is how I believe events may have unfolded:

Gladding buys the Sumner book while still with the US Revenue Service (1851, or later), writing his name inside to protect his property. After the passing of a few years, he joins the US Navy, taking his collection of navigational books with him. When the Southern states secede at the beginning of the Civil War, the loyal Southerner quits the navy (like so many other navy men at the time) and offers his services to the Confederacy.

Gladding gradually makes a name for himself running the Federal blockade in the famous Confederate schooner Parliament. *Still later, Gladding assumes command of the Rebel steamer* Reliance, *which is engaged in running cotton to international markets to earn badly needed money for an increasingly cash-strapped Confederate government.*

On July 21 or 22, 1862, Reliance *is pursued by* Huntsville, *but she is unable to outrun the faster navy vessel, forcing Gladding to surrender his ship or be blown out of the water. Rogers then seizes the Rebel ship, confiscating Gladding's papers, books, and probably his chronometer and stock of liquor. Rogers writes a note on the inside left cover of Gladding's* New Method *as a remembrance of the day he captured a Confederate ship.*

Rogers seems to have been rather lucky in capturing blockade-running vessels. He and *Huntsville* had taken the Confederate privateer *Beauregard* near Abaco on November 12, 1861, the British schooner *Agnes* carrying Rebel cotton and rosin through the blockade on July 16, 1862, and another

British schooner *Surprise* on March 13, 1863, off Charlotte Harbor, Florida, with a cargo of Confederate cotton bound for Havana.

Lieutenant Gladding, it seems, had less luck than his Northern adversary Rogers, and probably would not have missed losing his Sumner book—he died in a Federal prison more than a year after being caught by Rogers and *Huntsville*. Gladding was evidently a Mason, as it was that order that interred his remains in Northern soil. A short time later his remains were disinterred, transported to the front lines, and, under a flag of truce, turned over to Confederate forces for burial in the South.

How Gladding's book found its way to a used-book store in Lunenburg more than 140 years after the capture of *Reliance* is a mystery that is very likely to remain unsolved.

13

Maiden Voyage a Bummer

When a sailing vessel is successfully launched and she enters her watery abode for the first time, the owner, builder and probably the designer all secretly breathe a collective sigh of relief. She has survived her first test—she hasn't disintegrated upon entering the water and has actually managed to remain afloat. She has finally left the realm of the theoretical for the real world of wind and wave, where her maiden voyage will reveal to her captain and crew all her peculiarities and peccadilloes . . .

—J. GREGORY DILL

There comes a time in the lives of great personages when they feel compelled to erect a monument to their worldly accomplishments. For a modern VIP, this monument might take the form of a one-of-a-kind sailing yacht. But when King Gustavus Adolphus of Sweden ("Gus" to his friends at the sauna) approached the zenith of his political and military career in the seventeenth century, he chose to build the greatest warship the world had yet seen. She was to be named *Vasa*, for that illustrious royal household, and in 1625 Gus ordered her construction to help forge his dreams of Swedish military domination of Northern Europe. He even brought in Henrik Hyberson de Groot, a famous Dutch shipwright, to execute his vision. The ship not only was to be an efficient mobile killing machine, but—through the carving and gilding arts of imported Dutch and German craftsmen—was also to serve as a sumptuously decorated roving propaganda tool for a new and mighty Swedish Empire.

Even though De Groot died during her construction, *Vasa*'s launch went off without a hitch. She didn't fall apart when she hit the water, and she displaced the appropriate amount of briny to stay afloat—much to the delight of Peter de Groot, the younger brother of Henrik, who had taken charge of her final construction.

While she was still outfitting at dockside, Admiral Klas Fleming arrived to watch *Vasa* undergo stability testing. The "high-tech" testing procedure consisted of having thirty seamen run from the port to starboard rails, and back again, repeatedly. But after only three crossings of the deck the test was discontinued because the shiny new vessel was on the verge of capsizing at the dock. Fortunately Gus was abroad at the time, busy raping and pillaging Poland, so he didn't witness the test. In a nautical version of "The Emperor's New Clothes," no one wanted to send news to the impatient king that there might be just the tiniest problem with *Vasa*'s sea-keeping qualities.

By the tenth of August 1628, *Vasa* had become a veritable smorgasbord of firepower and fine art. She was stuffed with everything from munitions to meatballs and pikes to pickled herring, and finally ready to commence her maiden voyage. To mark that momentous event, one of her "great guns" was fired. At first only a few cat's paws teased the water's surface, and the great ark of art made slow forward progress. But the sound of *Vasa*'s celebratory gun must have awakened Nyord, the old Norse god of wind and sea, because less than a mile into her first voyage she was struck by a gust of wind that heeled her over. Immediately, before she could recover, a second, stronger gust slapped the great vessel down almost to her beam-ends. For what must have seemed an eternity, the captain and crew waited for *Vasa* to regain her composure. But she was incapable of righting herself. And to make matters worse, all of *Vasa*'s gun ports had been left open, and water quickly poured into the bowels of the ship, causing her to settle rapidly. Within minutes she disappeared below the surface. Tragically, *Vasa*'s Danish captain, Sofring Hansson, was unfamiliar with that ancient Swedish proverb: *Don't count your chickens until the hatches are closed.*

Today *Vasa* resides permanently within a special museum building in Stockholm, having been raised from her watery tomb and preserved (sort of) for posterity. Although a dismal failure as a fighting ship, she has finally managed to find her true niche—as a seventeenth-century objet d'art. Obese cherubs, Roman heroes, seductive mermaids, and rampant lions with attitudes stare back at visitors in all their former gilded, baroque glory. But for sailing enthusiasts the world over, *Vasa* will forever stand as a reminder of how *not* to begin a maiden voyage.

Bosun's Pipe—A Handy Guide

Good Boatswain, have care. Where's the Master? Play the men.

—ACT 1, SCENE 1, *THE TEMPEST* BY WILLIAM SHAKESPEARE

s a supernatural storm batters his ship, the frightened king of Naples pesters the harried ship's bosun, urging him to "play the men"—to call all hands on deck by playing his bosun's pipe. Later in the same scene the beleaguered bosun laments the noise and interference of the panicking landlubbers with the words, "A plague upon this howling: they are louder than the weather, or our office"— meaning that even the shrill squeals of his pipe can't be heard above the

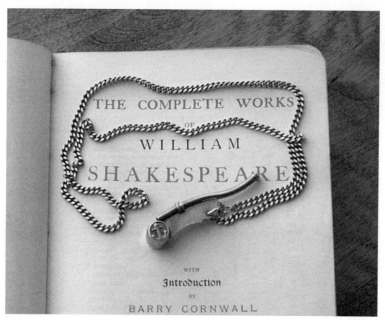

A bosun's pipe with neck chain. An early reference to the bosun's pipe appears in Shakespeare's play The Tempest. ©2005 by J. Gregory Dill

anxious cries. Such is the antiquity of that humble, quasi-musical instrument that has become synonymous with the office of ship's bosun.

Admiral Nimitz was greeted with the distinctive, high-pitched squeals of a bosun's pipe whenever he boarded his flagship during World War II, as was King Richard I when he stepped aboard his vessel before cruising off to the Crusades some seven centuries earlier. Captain Kirk was no stranger to the sounds of the bosun's pipe during his frequent materializations in the transporter room of the starship *Enterprise*, and even defeated Emperor Napoleon received a polite piped salute as he boarded HMS *Bellerophon* before being packed off by his British captors to exile on the island of St. Helena.

The bosun's pipe was developed as an effective communication tool for delivering instructions to ships' crews by means of a series of shrill notes capable of being heard anywhere in a vessel, or high above in the tops. During the noise of battle or in storm conditions when the human voice might become inaudible, the pipe's high-pitched renderings could be depended upon to punch a bosun's message through.

What exactly is a bosun's pipe? It's really little more (apologies to any offended bosuns) than a simple whistle, constructed of copper or brass, and maybe chrome- or silver-plated. Henry VIII's Lord High Admiral was in the habit of wearing something showier, a jewel-encrusted

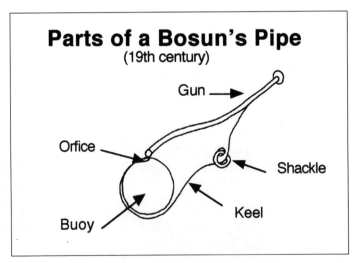

Parts of a bosun's pipe. ©2005 by J. Gregory Dill

gold bosun's pipe on a heavy gold chain, to proclaim his position as top Tudor tar. But this was hardly the kind of bauble blown by a burly bosun.

The main parts of the standard bosun's pipe bear suitably salty names (see diagram)—the *buoy*, the *keel*, the *shackle*, the *gun*, and the *orifice*. To play it, the pipe is held between the index finger and thumb, the latter being on or near the shackle. The side of the buoy rests against the palm of the hand, and the fingers close over the gun, buoy, and orifice so that the exit air may be throttled to the desired degree. Care must be taken that the fingers do not impinge upon the edge of the orifice in the buoy, or on the end of the gun nearest the buoy, as this will stifle all sound. A combination of tongue and finger movement, while blowing, produces distinct notes and trills.

The US Navy's *Bluejackets Manual* (1967) notes:

Even though there are loudspeaker and intercommunication systems on modern ships, the boatswain's pipe also is used for calling and passing the word.

Some calls identified in the manual are:

1) *Word to be passed*—Piped to command silence before passing an order or information.
2) *All hands*—Piped to call all hands' attention.
3) *Boat*—Piped to call away a boat; also to call a division or divisions to quarters.
4) *Call mates*—Piped by the boatswain to assemble his mates; also to arouse quick notice or attention from a working group.
5) *Mess gear*—Piped for mess gear.
6) *Piping the side*—Accompanies appropriate side honors. Signal that official personages are coming aboard [the president perhaps, or Bob Hope when he entertained the fleet].

It's interesting to speculate whether that old sailors' superstition about whistling aboard ship might have come about as a result of confusing the sound made by human lips with that made by the bosun's pipe. Pity the poor sailor whose thoughtlessly whistled ditty brought his off-watch messmates to battle stations. The unfortunate wretch would undoubtedly have been rudely told to *pipe down*, or be quiet—a call in the repertory of a piping bosun whose meaning has crept into contemporary language ashore.

Although playing of the bosun's pipe aboard ship has diminished in recent decades, most navies still employ the ancient instrument for ceremonial purposes—and if Gene Roddenberry got it right, the bosun's pipe might eventually see use beyond this world, on some intergalactic ship, traveling "where no man has gone before."

Duty and Honor, A Delicate Balance

A man has honor if he holds himself to an ideal of conduct though it is inconvenient, unprofitable or dangerous to do so.

—WALTER LIPPMANN

Walter Lippmann might have had career navy man William Henry Allen in mind when he penned the quote above. Allen, born in 1784 at Providence, Rhode Island, decided early in life to follow a career at sea, joining the fledgling US Navy in 1800 as a midshipman.

Later, as a lieutenant aboard the frigate USS *Chesapeake* in 1807, Allen proved his courage and dedication to his flag when *Chesapeake* was attacked by HMS *Leopard* for failing to submit to a British search for Royal Navy deserters aboard the US ship. Allen, using a glowing coal taken from the ship's galley fire and carried to the gun in his bare hands, fired the only gun available to reply to the savage British onslaught.

By 1812, America was at war with Britain, and Allen was in command of USS *Argus*, a brig-sloop of 250 tons. Allen's orders were crystal clear—hunt down and sink every British merchantman encountered near the coasts of Great Britain. Allen found the work personally distasteful, feeling he should be engaging Royal Navy ships and not helpless, unarmed civilian vessels.

While his sense of duty compelled him to destroy unarmed enemy freighters returning to Britain from her many overseas colonies, Allen's sense of honor induced him to find a way to avoid killing civilian crewmen and passengers aboard his victims. He balanced duty with a sense of fair play and allowed passengers and crews to escape safely with their personal possessions before destroying their ships. Those who reached shore recalled that Allen actually apologized to them before laying out their course to land. Always the gentleman, Allen was apparently moved to give his own deck coat to a freezing, nearly naked British seaman escaping in a lifeboat.

Despite his unorthodox approach to marine warfare, Allen and *Argus* were highly successful in destroying enemy tonnage, forcing Britain's Royal Navy to send every available vessel to sea in an effort to locate and rid their shores of *Argus* and "Gentleman Willie." Finally on August 14, 1814, HMS *Pelican* chanced upon *Argus* as she was standing to, allowing yet another merchantman's crew to escape danger before destroying her. The larger and more heavily armed *Pelican* delayed attacking *Argus* long enough to allow the intended victim's passengers and crew to escape danger. Ironically, *Pelican*'s crew gave Allen and his men three cheers for their chivalrous action before engaging the Yankee ship in battle.

After a furious engagement that left Allen with a severe leg wound and his small ship badly crippled, *Argus*'s standard was lowered, signifying defeat. Four days later, while being held in Plymouth prison, Allen died due to complications resulting from his leg having been amputated.

Allen was buried with full British military honors at Plymouth. His casket was carried through the streets accompanied by two companies of Royal Marines and a full honor guard, while some of those whose lives had been spared by the Yankee captain followed behind. Even merchants who had lost small fortunes to Allen's actions doffed their hats in respect. The city also took the extraordinary step of erecting a monument to Captain Allen inscribed with the words, HERE SLEEPS THE BRAVE—possibly the only memorial in any country to honor an enemy seaman.

16

Sea Cloud's *Eclectic Life*

L ike Bill Gates's mansion and Donald Trump's tower, millionaire financier Edward F. Hutton wanted his new yacht to symbolize his financial success. To that end, in 1930 Hutton ordered construction of an extravagant pleasure vessel as a wedding gift for his equally well-heeled wife, Marjorie Merriweather Post (of Post Grape-Nuts fame).

The 316-foot, four-masted bark initially slipped down the ways at the famous Krupp Germania Werft shipyard at Keil, Germany, on April 25, 1931, bearing the name *Hussar*. With cost no object, Krupp designers were instructed to install every cutting-edge convenience 1930s technology could offer. This included four auxiliary eight-hundred-horsepower diesel engines feeding power through an advanced electric transmission, for those times when the powerful guests invited aboard could not generate enough political wind to fill the bark's almost thirty-four thousand square feet of sail.

Electrical generators and the latest radio equipment ensured that VIPs would not suffer the privations normal life at sea offered regular sailors. Trim stabilizers were even installed to protect the delicate lubber constitutions of the rich and dainty who would be Hutton's guests. And because the ever-elegant Marjorie couldn't be expected to serve distinguished visitors hardtack and gruel, modern cooking and refrigeration equipment was also installed in *Hussar*'s galley. Marjorie even brought aboard a priceless collection of china that she proceeded to glue into display cabinets so it could be safely on show, even during a blow. By 1935 Marjorie had changed the name of the vessel to *Sea Cloud*, thinking possibly that the name *Hussar* was just a bit too lusty for the elegant bark.

A steady parade of kings, heads of state (including Franklin D. Roosevelt), crown princes, dictators, and other assorted 1930s luminaries attended Marjorie's formal floating dinner parties. After dining, guests might choose to saunter on deck in dinner jackets and gowns and, with glasses of champagne, toast one another on successfully roughing it at sea. When the sea's siren song finally failed to hold their interest any longer, the weary sailors might choose to retire to staterooms where, in the glowing comfort of marble fireplaces and leather armchairs, they could imagine themselves cruising in a Fifth Avenue apartment as they sipped brandy and examined the day's telegrams from home.

During World War II, Marjorie (by then Mrs. Joseph Davies) chartered *Sea Cloud* to the US government for the sum of one dollar per year. The vessel was initially employed as a weather ship on North Atlantic station, a duty *Sea Cloud* carried out while stripped of her masts. As the war continued, the ship was reassigned as a US Navy submarine spotter and was actually credited with assisting in the destruction of three German submarines (which were most likely built by the same Krupp shipyard that produced *Sea Cloud*).

Following the end of the war, *Sea Cloud* regained her masts, and the vessel returned to her luxurious prewar elegance. But by 1955 Marjorie had tired of her toy and sold the vessel to Rafael Trujillo, playboy dictator of the Dominican Republic. Following his death in 1961, *Sea Cloud* went into a period of decline in Santo Domingo Harbor.

After a couple of failed schemes to have the vessel make money, she was finally purchased by a German consortium in 1978 and returned to her original magnificence at the Krupp shipyard that had produced her. Today the restored *Sea Cloud* sails the ocean as a cruise ship, offering paying passengers a taste of life at sea as experienced by Marjorie Post and her pampered guests.

The Unfortunate Brig Phebe Ellen

Captain Robert Dill was a Master Mariner and a man of very strict religious convictions, whether at sea or ashore. When not abroad on a trading voyage in one of the family's two sailing vessels, Captain Dill assumed his responsibilities as an elder at the little Presbyterian church his grandfather had helped found at Londonderry, on the shores of the Bay of Fundy, in 1761.

So concerned was this seasoned seaman that Sunday be reserved for quiet reflection and worship that he initiated a petition to the governor of His Majesty's Province of Nova Scotia, requesting that the arrival time of Londonderry's Sunday mail coach from Halifax (bearing the Liverpool and Boston packet mails) be changed to a time well after church services had concluded. Much to Captain Robert's displeasure, and usually before the weekly sermon had begun, the first sounds of galloping hooves and rumbling coach wheels never failed to empty the humble seaside church of worshipers who evidently had a hankering for news of a more worldly nature.

Such displays by Captain Robert Dill to keep the Sabbath were not lost on his young son John, who joined his father at sea as cabin boy when only ten. When he was sixteen, during the American Civil War, John was already a veteran, having run the Union blockade of a Confederate port with his father in the family's smallest schooner, *Margaret Dill*. By 1870 John was an experienced twenty-three-year-old seaman and, like his father, had also obtained a Master Mariner certificate. By this time the family operated three trading vessels out of the Bay of Fundy—two schooners and a full-rigged, 182-ton brig christened *Phebe Ellen* for Captain Robert's youngest daughter. These vessels regularly sailed a triangular trading route, taking them from Nova Scotia to the West Indies and South America, then on to Britain and Europe, and finally back to Nova Scotia, carrying a variety of trade goods and cargo. But Captain Robert was beginning to grow tired of life at sea. He decided it was time to "swallow the anchor"—the old nautical term for retiring from the sea—and he began a new, low-stress career as Londonderry's postmaster. That decision propelled John into his first command, as captain of *Phebe Ellen*.

That John had inherited his father's strong inclination to keep Sunday as a day of rest seemed in little doubt, but those seamen who knew the young captain never felt he would deliberately endanger his vessel and crew because of his beliefs. Anyone who did not know him might find some of his actions strange for an experienced and respected seaman. Not surprising, then, was it that on November 26, 1871, a Sunday, *Phebe Ellen* was spotted in the distance by a perplexed Captain Colby of the steamer *Charlotta* near Seal Island, twelve nautical miles west of Cape Sable, Nova Scotia. *Charlotta*'s captain at first thought that some misfortune had overtaken the brig, since she was rolling about with all her sails furled to the yards, even though there was a brisk sailing breeze. Through his glass, Colby clearly observed that the brig's crew was all on deck, apparently in no distress. As everything aboard the brig appeared shipshape, Colby closed his glass and *Charlotta* steamed on her way. In this instance Captain John had simply decided that he could safely choose not to "work ship" on a Sunday. But just six weeks later his religious inclinations and the weather would conspire to seal the fates of himself and the crew of *Phebe Ellen*.

Saturday, January 6, 1872, found *Phebe Ellen* at the port of St. John, New Brunswick, taking on a cargo of shooks (oak barrel staves and headings) destined for Don Facundo Bacardi's rum distillery at Santiago de Cuba. David Dill, John's schoolmaster brother, had joined the brig at Saint John for the voyage south as acting second mate and navigator. Cargo loading was not completed until near midnight, and because the next day was Sunday, *Phebe Ellen* was not readied for sea until the following midnight, despite the fact that a favorable wind and tide on Sunday would have speeded the brig's safe exit from the Bay of Fundy.

So it was that *Phebe Ellen* did not slip her moorings until early Monday morning, January 8, on an incoming tide and falling barometer. The brisk northwesterly breeze pushing her on quickly blew into a gale. As the brig moved out into the rough water of the bay, frequent snow squalls enveloped her. She began to labor in the deteriorating conditions as snow and ice accumulation on her sails, masts, and spars quickly rendered the brig unstable. A short time later *Phebe Ellen* capsized.

Captain John, his brother David, and the other crewmen clung to the hull until *Phebe Ellen*'s deck load separated, at which time she righted herself, but not before her masts, spars, and rigging, as well as the deck-house, were torn away, as was the rudder. The men scrambled back onto the deck—all except the cook, a man named Vance. He lost his grip, fell overboard, and was quickly swept from sight in the churning waters. The brig was now totally out of control and driving steadily on in a hurricane wind toward the southwest coast of Nova Scotia.

Hours later *Phebe Ellen*'s end came when she drove upon a ledge at Youngs Cove. The men were thoroughly soaked and nearly frozen. They had not been able to retrieve dry clothing from belowdecks or prepare hot food, because the galley and crew's quarters were underwater. Captain John ordered his suffering crew to help him release the bow anchor in the hope it might hold the brig's present position on the ledge long enough for the men to get ashore. The anchor was deployed, but the chain soon parted under the load, and *Phebe Ellen* worked on the ledge until she began to break up.

In the end only three of the eight men aboard survived the wreck. Captain John Dill was crushed between colliding ice pans as he tried to

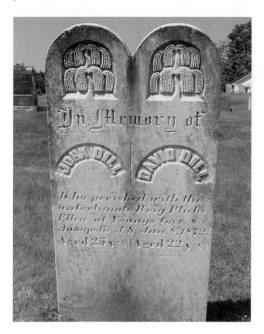

This headstone documents the sad fate of brothers John and David Dill, captain and second mate of the unfortunate brig Phebe Ellen.
©2004 by J. Gregory Dill

swim ashore with a line. David and two crewmen died of hypothermia on the wreck before they could be rescued. Old Captain Robert Dill in Londonderry received the following cryptic telegram advising him of the disaster:

> BRIG PHEBE ELLEN HERE YOUNG'S COVE—CAPTAIN AND COOK LOST—THREE MEN DEAD—THREE LIVING.

Devastated by the news of the loss of his son, Robert Dill collapsed clutching the telegram. Only later did he learn that his other son, David, had also died on the wreck—both victims of the weather and perhaps an overly strict observance of Sabbath.

POSTSCRIPT: THE TALE OF *PHEBE ELLEN*'S CHRONOMETER

In his grief at the deaths of his two sons and other crew in the loss of his brig *Phebe Ellen*, Captain Robert Dill appointed his good friend Captain P. D. Fletcher to act as his agent at the wreck scene. While securing what could be salvaged of *Phebe Ellen*'s cargo, Fletcher learned that the brig's chronometer had actually survived the wreck and had been found, its wooden case still securely screwed to a cabin table that had floated free from *Phebe Ellen*'s destroyed deckhouse. Chronometers were indispensable and expensive navigational instruments used in determining a ship's longitude at sea. Though likely damaged by seawater, the valuable instrument might be repaired and used again. When Captain Fletcher further inquired after the navigational timepiece, he discovered it had been taken from the beach by one Isaiah Sabine who, after keeping it in his possession for forty-eight hours, had taken it to a clock maker named Sancton in the nearby community of Bridgetown. When Fletcher visited the clock maker, Sancton told him that he had advised Sabine that if the chronometer was insured, he (Sabine) would be entitled to twenty dollars for recovering it, and he (Sancton) would charge ten dollars for safely storing it. Sancton said he advised Mr. Sabine that if it was not insured, he should ask only ten dollars from the owner of the brig, and he himself would ask only five dollars for storing it.

Enraged at Sancton's gall, Fletcher insisted that the clock maker turn over the navigational timepiece immediately, as he was the duly appointed agent for the wreck. Sancton refused, quickly removing the chronometer and locking it in a room at the back of his shop.

Captain Fletcher was only able to obtain the chronometer by hiring a local lawyer, who promptly advised the clock maker by letter to deliver the timepiece at once or risk being charged with theft from a wreck—a hanging offense at the time. Sancton took the ten dollars and grudgingly handed over the chronometer, which Fletcher then delivered to old Captain Dill at Londonderry. The chronometer was restored to working condition and, although no longer accurate enough for navigation, it ticked out its days in the little Presbyterian church attended by the Dill family—a memorial to the tragedy and loss of the unfortunate brig *Phebe Ellen.*

An Unlikely U-boat Hunter

Tucked into the north coast of Cuba, a few miles east of Havana's harbor entrance, lies the unassuming little fishing port of Coji-mar. A casual visitor to the town will be pleasantly surprised to find the locals politely curious about his or her presence in their friendly community, unlike the reception the same visitor might expect from panhandlers and street hustlers in tourist-ridden parts of Old Havana, only a few minutes away by car.

Down near the water's edge two structures immediately take the visitor's eye. The first, resembling a pirate-themed fast-food franchise, is a small rectangular stone fort of some antiquity commanding the mouth

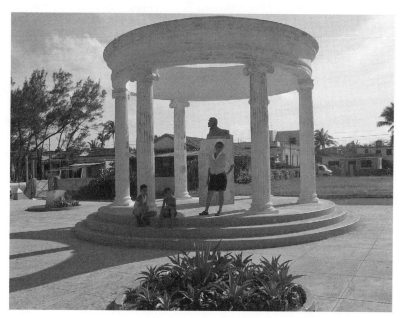

The fishermen of the port of Cojimar, Cuba, erected this memorial to Ernest Hemingway to honor the author's winning of the Nobel Prize for his novella The Old Man and the Sea. ©2005 by J. Gregory Dill

of the Cojimar River. With 240-year-old repairs to the damaged walls of the fort still plainly visible, travelers might expect the building to harbor some romantic tale of corsairs and Spanish gold that would make a stop at this otherwise unremarkable backwater worthwhile. In fact there is a tale—one of a spirited and bloody hour-long firefight between the fort's Spanish defenders and a small Royal Navy frigate, HMS *Dragon*, which entered the mouth of the river on June 7, 1762, in support of a massive British attack on Havana. But that's another story.

For most visitors, the principal reason to visit Cojimar is to view the unusual monument erected in the small plaza bordering the fort. That monument, built with money raised by local fishermen, celebrates the memory of a famous American who was locally well respected as a friend—writer Ernest Hemingway. Here in Cojimar, Hemingway found the poor but tenacious fishermen who collectively became the inspiration for the stubborn and grizzled Santiago, star of the Nobel Prize–winning novella *The Old Man and the Sea*. It was here, too, that Hemingway chose to keep his beloved fishing yacht and where he spent many enjoyable hours with the locals at La Terraza Bar and Restaurant, drinking and listening to the fishermen's experiences at sea.

Fishing had long been a pleasant pastime for Hemingway. So when the editor of *Esquire* magazine sent the author a cash advance for a planned series of articles to be written in 1934, Hemingway promptly used part of the money to order a yacht to satisfy his growing passion for bluewater fishing. Wheeler Shipyard of New York undertook to custom-build a motor launch for the novelist, using its thirty-eight-foot "Playmate" model as a starting point for the special order. With a twelve-foot beam and drawing less than four feet of water, this was to be a serious boat for marlin fishing in Gulf Stream waters. She was stoutly built of cedar and white oak, and Hemingway specified that she was to have large-capacity fuel tanks to feed her 110-horsepower Chrysler marine engine for extended cruising and fishing expeditions. She was also to have a flying bridge sufficiently high to allow an unrestricted view in all directions, and with enough room below to comfortably accommodate up to six guests. The author christened his beautiful yacht *Pilar*, a name he would later give to a female character in his novel *For Whom the Bell Tolls*.

Hemingway moved to Cuba on the eve of World War II, taking *Pilar* with him and arranging to have her conveniently berthed at Cojimar

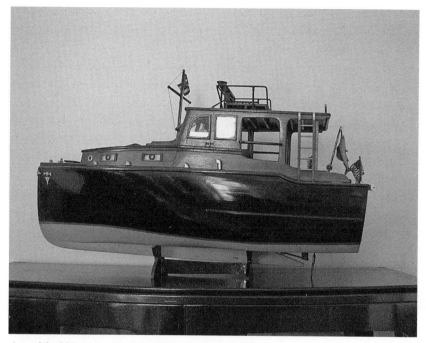

A model of Hemingway's beloved yacht Pilar. ©2005 by J. Gregory Dill

while he and his future wife, journalist Martha Gellhorn, ensconced themselves at a secluded fifteen-acre villa several miles away called Finca Vigia. Once settled, Hemingway entered into a regimen of writing, marlin fishing with his beloved *Pilar*, and imbibing with his buddies at La Bodeguita and El Floridita bars in Havana and La Terraza in Cojimar. But by May 1942 Papa's happy, halcyon days were destined to undergo some modification, thanks in part to Karl Donitz, grand admiral of Germany's U-boat fleet.

Admiral Donitz had authorized Operation Drumbeat (*Paukenschlag*) to begin the first day of May, unleashing an unprecedented submarine assault on North American shipping. Drumbeat included specific authorization for two submarines to take up station and commence search-and-destroy operations against Allied shipping in the Gulf of Mexico and the heavily navigated Bahama Channel, waters that included some of Hemingway's favorite fishing areas. On May 4 Korvettenkapitan Harro Schacht of *U-507* sent the first Allied casualty to the bottom off Key West, Florida— the 2,686-ton freighter *Norlindo*. This event ushered in a monthlong sinking spree by U-boats that saw almost a freighter a day dispatched to the seafloor and fear struck into merchant sailors' hearts at US, Bahamian, and Cuban ports.

With few Allied aircraft or ships to intervene, the subs' commanders often chose to surface beside smaller, unsuspecting freighters, which would then be attacked and sunk using deck guns only, saving expensive torpedoes for larger and more deserving marine game. The U-boat crews had even begun playing pirate, scavenging fresh water, food, liquor, and tobacco from small pleasure craft and fishing boats such as those that ventured out of Cojimar daily. News of these unchallenged raids and sinkings by the Germans began to appear regularly on the front pages of Havana papers and became the most popular topic of conversation among Hemingway and friends at the bar of La Terraza in Cojimar.

The author's irrepressible hunting instincts very quickly became irreversibly aroused. Hemingway found it impossible to resist the call of the hunt and decided to hit back at the Nazi raiders with an aggressive, if somewhat fanciful, plan to fit out *Pilar* as a submarine hunter-killer. Perhaps he thought a U-boat Korvettenkapitan's cap might make a distinctive addition to the collection of mounted safari trophies adorning the walls at Finca Vigia. The author knew Spruille Braden, US ambassador to Cuba, and enlisted Braden's assistance in bringing his scheme to fruition. Braden was a genuine fan of Hemingway's writing and arranged for delivery of weaponry to Cojimar for *Pilar*, including two .50-caliber machine guns and crates of hand grenades. Well stocked with ammunition, drinking buddies, and plenty of ice and rum for Papa's favorite libations, daiquiris and mojitos, *Pilar* began her brave excursions past the little square fort at the mouth of the Cojimar River, then out into the dangerous Bahama Channel to hunt for brazen Nazi prey.

How exactly this classic wooden sportfishing craft was supposed to successfully attack and destroy a surfaced submarine has remained a bit of a mystery. Presumably, as a sub closed on *Pilar*, the spectacle of her tipsy crew uncovering machine guns would produce paroxysms of laughter among the submariners, incapacitating them long enough for *Pilar*'s crew to fumble a grenade or two through the open hatch of the sub's conning tower. But *Pilar* would never have had a serious chance of engaging a surfaced submarine. No U-boat commander would have approached any surface craft without having his boat's deck gun loaded, manned, and trained on the vessel of interest—U-boat commanders had learned that hard lesson very well during World War I. Had *Pilar* been unfortunate enough to encounter her intended prey, an armed German boarding party would first have been dispatched to the yacht in an inflatable boat while the surfaced submarine remained a safe distance off. The sub would have approached *Pilar* only after the boarding party signaled they had taken possession of the boat. The sub's gun could easily have reduced *Pilar* to matchsticks with one shot from two hundred yards at the first sign of any hostile action.

But there were other potentially grave consequences for the author once he had guided *Pilar* out of the safety of Cojimar. Even if Havana had not been rife with Nazi spies gathering intelligence on ship movements and passing the same to the German high command, a chance encounter between Hemingway and a U-boat might have exposed the author to a possibility no one involved in the oddball scheme seems to have considered—Hemingway's capture by a U-boat crew. Imagine the coup to be scored by Dr. Joseph Goebbels, Nazi propaganda chief, had

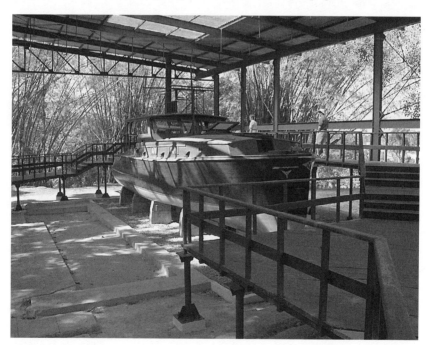

Pilar *lies safe under cover at Hemingway's former villa near Havana.*
©2005 by J. Gregory Dill

he been able to parade Papa before the Third Reich's news media. Public display before newsreel cameras of a captured US literary luminary like Ernest Hemingway might have proven a significant blow to American morale.

After conducting numerous unsuccessful missions out of Cojimar with *Pilar* during 1942–43, Ernest Hemingway and his crew probably did not appreciate how fortunate they had been in having failed to confront and engage even one enemy U-boat—fortuitous also for those Hemingway fans who enjoy reading Papa's later fiction. But the dangerous and futile patrols did serve a practical purpose after all, providing a source of raw material that would later be woven into the plot of Hemingway's popular, posthumously published novel, *Islands in the Stream.*

Ernest Hemingway eventually left Cuba in 1960 after Fidel Castro came to power. The author boarded up his villa and gave the (by then) severely deteriorated *Pilar* to his longtime mate and Cojimar friend, Gregorio Fuentes. Today Finca Vigia is a museum celebrating the memory of Papa's years in Cuba, and *Pilar* has been restored and put on permanent display on the estate's grounds, under a protective roof, minus her wartime machine guns, a remembrance of Papa's heroic, if ill-conceived, hunting safaris from the quiet little fishing port of Cojimar on the north coast of Cuba, searching for that most cunning and elusive of all trophy fish—the German U-boat.

19

Dr. Jekyll and Captain Hyde

In the field of ocean navigation, there may be no greater enigma than Captain William Dampier. Dampier was a consummate navigator, cartographer, explorer, zoologist, botanist, artist, author, lecturer, drug runner, slaver, and pirate. He was equally at home swinging a cutlass beside bloodthirsty crewmates on the Spanish Main as he was lecturing on his botanical and geographic discoveries before genteel scholars in London salons. And by the end of his life Dampier had undertaken three circumnavigations of the globe, making him one of the most traveled men of the seventeenth and early eighteenth centuries.

Born in England in 1652, Dampier began his years at sea by fishing on Newfoundland's Grand Banks in the 1670s; by 1683 the experienced seaman was a member of the crew of the infamous pirate vessel *Bachelor's Delight*. Dampier's new home was a former Danish vessel of thirty-six guns converted by her pirate crew to a dangerous and highly effective vessel for attacking fat merchantmen carrying any cargo and flying any flag. But Dampier seems to have chosen not to participate in the debauched revels of his peers whenever they returned to land to celebrate the taking of some rich prize, or after having successfully looted a coastal town. While his mates were drinking and whoring, Dampier would wander off with his charcoal, pencils, and drawing paper to study and record the local flora and fauna. When he tired of documenting the nesting habits of exotic birds, he might then choose to survey and map the coast or study and record the peculiarities of local winds and tidal variations. So observant was he that he later published a book titled *Discourse of Winds, Breezes, Storms, Tides, and Currents of the Torrid Zone*—a notable sailing guide that greatly advanced the knowledge of his fellow navigators.

Dampier completed his first circumnavigation on September 16, 1691, returning to England broke but with his writings, maps, drawings, and a collection of items gathered during his travels. During the next six years he made a tenuous living lecturing on the curiosities he had collected and recorded during his voyage. In 1697 Dampier published a hugely successful book recounting his exploits and discoveries called *A New Voyage Round the World*. The overwhelming success of the book brought him an offer from the Admiralty to command HMS *Roebuck* for the purpose of conducting a voyage of discovery to the Far East. Unfortunately Dampier's inability to interact effectively with his officers in a reasonable manner revealed him to be an unskilled and ill-suited commander. When *Roebuck* arrived back in England, Dampier was relieved of command and court-martialed.

On Dampier's third circumnavigation he acted as pilot—a position more suited to his testy personality. It was during this voyage with Captain Woodes Rodgers that Dampier's ship stopped at the island of Juan Fernandez off the Pacific coast of South America, where his ship rescued a stranded seaman named Alexander Selkirk—the seaman who would become the model for Daniel Defoe's castaway, Robinson Crusoe.

Dampier was obviously not a pirate in the sense of Edward (Blackbeard) Teach or William Kidd. But he was chameleon-like, being a scholarly Dr. Jekyll one minute and an infamous Captain Hyde the next, the latter especially while in command of a vessel. When he died in meager circumstances in 1715, few people other than his contemporaries in the business of ocean navigation could imagine how much Dampier's published books would assist future marine explorers and scientists such as Captain James Cook and Charles Darwin in their famous voyages of discovery. In fact, William Dampier's writings would eventually be key elements in forming the foundations of the modern sciences of hydrography, botany, and zoology.

Tectonic Tremblings That Trashed a Town

. . . boatmen still assert that on stormy evenings one may hear the tolling of Port Royal's cathedral bell, lying fathoms deep beneath the waves.

—HARRY A. FRANCK

The morning of June 7, 1692, dawned bright and humid with not a hint of a sea breeze or the faintest suggestion that a disaster of biblical proportions was about to befall the eight thousand citizens of Port Royal, Jamaica.

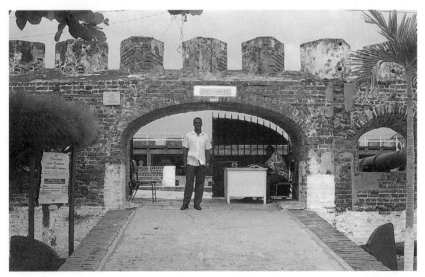

Although it did sink into the ground almost three feet during the 1692 earthquake and subsequent tsunami, Port Royal's Fort Charles was miraculously spared destruction. ©2004 by J. Gregory Dill

Here, in the town where profit and the pursuit of pleasure were paramount, aging buccaneers lived out their declining years in wealthy debauched ease while merchants made fortunes in the slave and sugar trades, or in victualing Royal Navy vessels. Even brothel owners, catering to seamen from the hundred or more merchant vessels constantly in the harbor, could expect to retire back in England where they might hope to live as well as any duke or duchess.

Port Royal was a key trade link in a cyclical marine route connecting England with the English settlements of St. Johns, Boston, and Jamestown. Port Royal unabashedly displayed the fruits of sea-born wealth in its elegant, well-appointed homes and public buildings. Wealthy citizens employed slaves or indentured servants to run their households and brought out tutors from England to give their children first-class educations. But even with its wealth and sophistication, the town could not hide its lawless nature, having taken on what might now best be described as a kind of Wild West/Key West flavor, with a little Central Park West thrown in for good measure. Arguments fostered by drink at the town's plentiful and always open alehouses and taverns tended to end in street confrontations where fists, pistols, and swords settled grudges with frequent and swift finality.

Nowhere in this wickedest of English colonial port towns could one find the puritanical angst and religious navel gazing rife up north in the commonwealth of Massachusetts, where in just three days' time condemned witch Bridget Bishop would be executed for "crimes" that would hardly raise an eyebrow in Port Royal. Life was good for the inhabitants of Jamaica's capital, and they had no good reason to expect that the town's prosperity would not continue as it had every year since England had captured the port from Spain in 1655.

The earthquake began just before noon, as noted by the Reverend Dr. Emmanuel Heath, who witnessed and survived the disaster. Heath wrote the following in a letter to England on June 19 from his temporary home aboard the sloop *Granada* anchored in Port Royal Harbor. Interestingly, the good clergyman's tale reveals he was having a few drinks with a friend at one of those numerous taverns when the earthquake began:

When I first felt ye Earth Quake I wondered what was ye matter hearing a great humming noise and finding ye earth playing under my feet.

Heath's three-page letter describes how he got out of the building without injury, then continues:

... as I made my way towards it [the fort] ye Earth opened and swallowed up many People before my face, and ye Sea I saw come mounting in over ye wall . . . and the destruction was very sudden and surprising, it being over in 4 minutes: multitudes were killed by the falling of houses, multitudes both of men and houses were swallowed up by ye gaping Earth, and many others were swept away by ye inundation [what we would now describe as an earthquake-induced tsunami].

Heath's letter concludes:

Tis a sad spectacle to see ye whole Harbour covered with dead floating carcases, with ye ruins of houses and wraks of goods, but ye smell is worse.

HMS *Swan*, a Fifth Rate naval vessel that was in the process of being careened (having her bottom scraped) when the quake began, was picked up by the wall of harbor water rushing in to replace the large portion of the town that had slid into the sea. *Swan* was literally thrown down upon some damaged homes, while other ships were torn from their mooring lines to drift ashore or out to sea. When the quake ended, less than 10 percent of the town's buildings were left standing, and two thousand citizens were dead.

Port Royal's glory days never returned after the earthquake of 1692. Many of the town's survivors left, and the Royal Navy moved most of its operations to the new and safer port of Kingston, a short distance away. Today Port Royal is little more than a sleepy fishing village. Only the port's old Fort Charles and a few tombstones remain to tell the tale.

When I visited the site in 2004 I found a tombstone belonging to Lewis Galdy, a citizen of Port Royal at the time of the 1692 quake. Galdy was evidently a man of exceptional luck. He actually survived the earthquake to live another forty-seven years. His tombstone epitaph recalls his earthquake ordeal:

Here lyes the Body of Lewis Galdy Esq. who departed this Life at Port Royal the 22d December 1739 Aged 80. He was Born at Montpeltier in France but left that Country for his Religion &

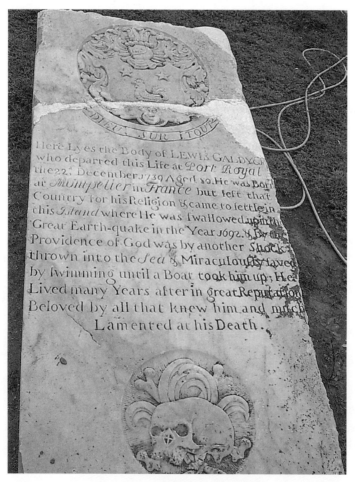

Lewis Galdy's tombstone tells of this gentleman's luck in surviving the Port Royal earthquake. ©2004 by J. Gregory Dill came to settle in this Island where He was swallowed up in the Great Earth-quake in the year 1692 & by the Providence of God was by another Shock thrown into the Sea & Miraculously saved by swimming until a Boat took him up.

Before leaving Port Royal I did listen at the water's edge for that ghostly tolling bell of the old cathedral fathoms below the surface, but could hear only the cries of gulls circling a boat returning from a day of fishing. Divers, as it turns out, had recovered the bell from the depths years before.

A Nonacademic Look at Helm History

The continual sight of the fiend shapes before me, caper-
ing half in smoke and half in fire, these at last begat kindred
visions in my soul, so soon as I began to yield to that unaccountable
drowsiness which ever would come over me at a midnight helm.

—*MOBY DICK* BY HERMAN MELVILLE

Had contemplation of that damned white whale not entirely
dominated his thoughts while at *Pequod*'s helm, Herman
Melville's sailor-schoolteacher Ishmael might have directed
his mind to more fruitful pursuits—like authoring a much-needed text
on the history and evolution of the marine steering apparatus under
his control.

Unfortunately, knowledge of the earliest methods for guiding vessels on water is either nonexistent or shadowy at best. Meager glimpses
into the subject have come from artistic details in marine scenes from
Egyptian burial chamber murals, Chinese rice paper paintings, Grecian
pottery, and Roman bathhouse mosaics, or somewhat more reliably
from underwater examinations of a limited number of well-preserved
ancient shipwrecks.

We do know that somewhere between five and six thousand years
ago watercraft of reed construction began appearing on Egypt's Nile,
powered by oars, and later by solitary sails. A steering oar (or sometimes
two) was used to direct a vessel's course and consisted of a flat piece of
wood attached to a sturdy wooden shaft or pole and lashed to the side
of a vessel's stern. Later Greek and Roman vessels used similar oared
steering to navigate.

While boatbuilding technology steadily advanced during the next few
thousand years, the humble steering oar remained virtually unchanged,

even into the early Viking era of the tenth century. The Vikings called the Nordic version of the steering oar a *styribord* or steering board. Incidentally, the Viking steering oar was mounted on the right side of the stern—the *styribord* side—a word that later linguistically morphed into the English nautical term *starboard.*

As ship size grew and forces acting on steering oars increased, an additional piece of wood (a long bar or handle) was fastened near the top of the steering oar shaft. This handle, the forerunner of the tiller, could be swung horizontally to provide leverage advantage to ease steering loads for the helmsman. Bigger craft required a longer handle so that more than one man might be brought to bear to keep the vessel under control, especially when conditions deteriorated. In really heavy weather the steering oar might spend a good deal of time out of the water, resulting in loss of steering control.

About the time King Richard I was setting sail to begin his Middle Eastern military adventures (1190 CE), some bright Teutonic shipwright living on the shores of the Baltic began building a traditional local vessel known as a Cog—traditional except for some highly unique steering modifications. The builder had eliminated the steering oar's limitations by attaching a hinged steering board directly to the sternpost of the Cog. He still employed a tiller, but it was now attached to the head of the steering board so that it could be turned from side to side to direct steering board movement about a vertical axis. Mounted on the centerline of the ship, and low down so that it would always remain in the water, the newly positioned steering board improved steering response dramatically.

In the early fourteenth century, castle-like structures began to be installed on decks of fighting ships, resulting in the obscuring of the helmsman's view forward. This necessitated raising the helmsman's position to a higher vantage point. To control the tiller from his newly elevated position, a movable vertical shaft was installed, attached by a yoke to the tiller to transmit the helmsman's left and right steering movements into horizontal tiller deflections. This new shaft was called a whipstaff, quite possibly because of its potential to soundly thrash any inattentive helmsman during heavy weather.

By the late seventeenth century the word *rudder* had replaced *steering board.* Vessels were now approaching mega size, making their management at sea decidedly more difficult from a navigational point of view. Adapting a whipstaff to increasingly larger rudder-tiller combinations proved impractical, a situation that precipitated the next major steering innovation found today on every large ship. An anonymous Englishman devised a clever steering arrangement to control rudder movement (via the tiller) using blocks and tackle actuated by a rotating drum attached to a steering wheel. This device greatly improved mechanical advantage and allowed more precise incremental rudder positioning by a single helmsman, in moderate weather.

Fortunately, the anonymous developer of this wheeled steering revelation was able to construct a working version of his idea, a move that must have exposed him to much ridicule and scathing comment by

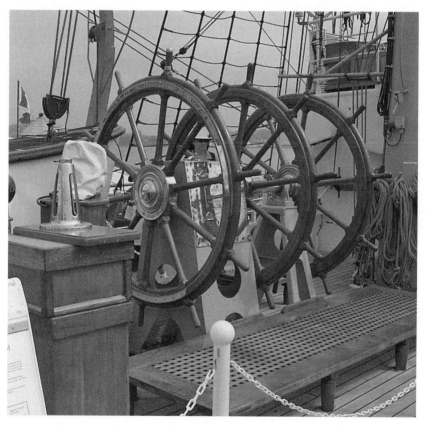

Three wheels, no waiting! The main helm of the US Coast Guard Eagle.
©2003 by J. Gregory Dill

peers who would have thought him completely mad. Had he chosen to take the easy course and flee from the criticism of his fellow seamen, perhaps by signing aboard a departing whaling ship, he might have squandered his creative mind standing nightly helm watches, like Herman Melville's Ishmael—obsessing about some evil albino cetacean.

The World's Most-Masted Schooner

When she slipped down the ways at the Fore River Ship and Engine Building Company in Quincy, Massachusetts, the $258,000 schooner *Thomas W. Lawson* was the only sailing vessel of her type in the world. That was July 10, 1902, and Coastwise Transportation Company officials who had ordered her construction more than a year earlier were on hand to watch her keel kiss salt water for the first time. They were quite confident that the new vessel's appearance on the shipping scene would not only silence the death knell for sail-powered ships, but also ring in a profitable new century for the company and its shareholders.

It was not the size of *Lawson* that made her unique, although her 380-foot length and her 5,216 gross registered tonnage were certainly impressive figures for a schooner. Nor was the fact that her hull was made of steel plate her main claim to fame. What singled out *Lawson* for special attention was the fact that she carried seven masts, suggesting that a whole forest ecosystem somewhere in the Maine woods must have been put to the saw and ax so that this behemoth might move upon the seas.

While finishing touches were being made to the distinctive ship, old seamen lined the quayside to behold the ultramodern *Lawson*, shaking their heads in disbelief and longing for the sailing days of their youth when ship spotting had been decidedly less difficult. How would they name all those masts—fore, main, and another one, and another one, and another one, and another one, and finally mizzen? And were all those steam-powered winches on her deck really necessary for sail handling? As it turned out, the winches were absolutely vital because *Lawson* carried an incredible twenty-five sails in all—seven gaff sails, seven topsails, six staysails, and five jibs—for a total sail area of more than 43,000 square feet. This mass of canvas weighed nearly eighteen tons dry, and when wet would make the vessel unstable and extremely difficult to handle in any kind of sea, so that she would never instill confidence in those who sailed her.

Lawson spent her first four years as a successful coal freighter before being modified in 1907 by Newport Shipbuilding and Dry Dock Company to carry bulk oil. Later that same year, on December 13—Friday the Thirteenth as it happened—she found herself unable to weather the Scilly Islands off the southwest coast of England. *Lawson*'s crew made preparations to anchor, but that evening a link in her anchor chain failed during a heavy blow. The chain parted and the ship drifted onto the rocks, taking the lives of thirteen of her crew and causing the total loss of the vessel.

Lawson was remarkable for being the first and last seven-masted schooner ever constructed. She did make money for her owners but was expensive to maintain and operate. In hindsight, it was fortunate that her designer, Bowdoin B. Crowninshield, opted not to go with his initial 1901 proposal for the ship. That plan called for a more costly four-hundred-foot, *eight*-masted design.

Unfortunate Times before the Mast

I t's 1914—the eve of World War I. You've come on deck early, before your anchor watch begins, to sip your coffee and survey the harbor in the fading light. Off the port rail you spot a square-rigged merchant vessel quietly getting under way, little changed in appearance from her nineteenth-century kin. Moments later you glance across the starboard rail to see a turbine-powered naval cruiser, billowing clouds of black smoke and bristling with the latest weaponry, entering the harbor in company with one of those new naval curiosities—the stealthy submarine.

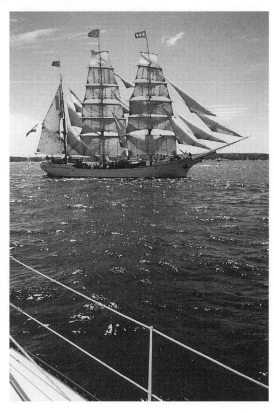

Unlike many of her unlucky contemporaries, the beautiful Hamburg-built bark Europa *(launched 1911) safely weathered two world wars to sail sedately into the twenty-first century.*
©2003 by J. Gregory Dill

Such visual ironies were common for sailors just prior to World War I. But the incongruity of unarmed, wind-powered vessels becoming the prey of modern high-speed naval ships could never have been fully comprehended by observant sailors, until hostilities began.

In his book *The Battle of the Falkland Islands; Before and After*, Commander H. Spencer-Cooper notes one such irony as hostilities commenced between British and German battle cruisers on December 8, 1914:

> . . . a full-rigged sailing ship appeared on the port hand of our battle cruisers; she was painted white, and her sails were shining as if bleached in the bright sunlight—so close was she that the Admiral was forced to alter his course to pass a couple of miles clear of her, so that the enemy's shell ricocheting should not hit her.

The sailing ship that had wandered into the middle of this naval engagement was the Norwegian full-rigged ship *Fairport*, en route from Chile to Norway. *Fairport* managed to run the gauntlet none the worse for her captain's navigational blunder—her crew most likely unaware that war had begun during their passage 'round the Horn.

George Hanks, a sick bay attendant aboard HMS *Carnarvon,* spotted another sailing vessel the same day not far from *Fairport*'s course line. In his diary Hanks recorded:

> About 3 p.m. a big sailing ship appears on the horizon and no doubt but what those on board her had a magnificent view of the battle just as it was at its zenith. (This unidentified vessel too was lucky to have escaped harm.)

American vessels were initially spared naval harassment, thanks to the US government policy of neutrality. But on January 27, 1915, while sailing off the Brazilian coast, Captain H. H. Kiehne of the 3,374-ton steel-built American bark *William P. Frye* (launched at Bath, Maine, 1901) was about to learn that being from a neutral country didn't count for much. The German armed cruiser *Prinz Eitel Friedrich* quickly overhauled *Frye* en route from Seattle to England with a cargo of wheat. Commander Max Thierichens of *Friedrich* ordered Kiehne to stop and prepare to receive a boarding party. When the Germans found *Frye* carrying "contraband" wheat bound for England, Thierichens demanded that Kiehne commence dumping his cargo. However, unloading progressed too slowly for the impatient German. Thierichens ordered Kiehne and his crew to come aboard *Friedrich* while a demolition team prepared their bark and her remaining cargo for destruction. *Frye* was sunk with a dynamite charge, gaining for the vessel the dubious honor of being the first American marine casualty of World War I.

Large vessels were not the only sail-powered victims of the war, however. On August 30, 1918, the 136-ton Lunenburg fishing schooner *Potentate* was proceeding home from the Grand Banks of Newfoundland. Captain Fred Gerhardt (a descendant of eighteenth-century German settlers at Lunenburg, Nova Scotia) was pleased with his catch—fourteen hundred quintals (140,000 pounds) of cod. As *Potentate* left the banks, fog engulfed the schooner. All was quiet, until an officious, heavily accented voice boomed through the mist:

Heave your ship to, and lower your sails!

When Gerhardt came topside to investigate, he found a surfaced German U-boat a short distance off *Potentate*'s beam. The same insistent voice ordered the Lunenburg captain to lower a dory and come aboard the submarine, where he and his two oarsmen were informed by the sub commander that their schooner would be sunk because it was, as the German said, "helping to feed America." After being held for two hours Gerhardt heard a muffled explosion. *Potentate* was "sent below" with a charge of dynamite, but not before the remaining crew on the schooner had been allowed to lower their dories, filled with belongings, food, and water. The commander offered Gerhardt and his men an apology for having destroyed their means of livelihood, in German, before setting them free in their dories. The commander threw Gerhardt a loaf of rye bread and a cask of water, and gave him a course to steer for the Newfoundland coast. *Potentate*'s captain and crew eventually arrived safely at St. Johns, Newfoundland.

Between August and September 1918 U-boats destroyed nine fishing schooners near the Grand Banks—unfortunate for their Canadian and American shareholders, given that hostilities with Germany would cease in November, just weeks later.

The exact number of vintage sailing ships lost to hostile action during those dangerous years will likely never be known.

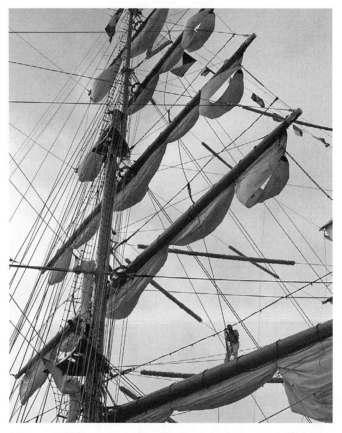

Life at sea for those manning sailing vessels during World War I was difficult and dangerous enough without having the additional worry of being shot at. ©2004 by J. Gregory Dill

24

Admiral Yi's Kobuksun

Like most world capitals, the city of Seoul in South Korea has its share of monuments to past national heroes. One of the most prominent is that of Admiral Yi Sun Shin (1545–1598), the most celebrated hero of his country.

Yi was a man of remarkable abilities. He was loyal and moralistic, and imbued with a George Washington–like patriotic fervor, a Lord Nelson–like tactical naval genius, and native intelligence. Yi was trained as a classical scholar and poet, but eventually entered the service of his king and country as a military man.

In 1592 (about the time William Shakespeare was writing *Richard III*), a hostile Japanese fleet made a surprise and unprovoked attack on Korea's coast. After years of peace and internal corruption, surprised and disorganized Korean defense forces were ill prepared to fend off the Japanese intrusion.

Yi, as a sector commander of coastal defense, designed a radically new vessel called a *kobuksun,* or turtle boat, and trained crews to man his strange craft and engage the massive Japanese fleet. Yi's boat design looked surprisingly like the *Merrimac* or *Monitor* of America's Civil War, 270 years into the future. The *kobuksun* design produced a shallow-draft vessel, armed with twenty-four medium guns and powered by oarsmen. A protective, rounded roof deck constructed of thin iron gave the boat a turtle-like appearance. The roof or weather deck was studded with iron spikes and sharpened blades to hinder enemy boarding attempts. At the height of the struggle with the Japanese, Korea had been able to construct only twelve turtle boats to oppose hundreds of armed Japanese vessels.

The most unusual aspect of Yi's vessel was the large dragon's head mounted on the bow, Viking fashion. But the head was more than simply decorative. As Yi's turtle boats approached the main Japanese sea force from downwind, sulfur fires were ignited in special burners within the boat, creating choking fumes that were ducted through the dragon's mouth to drift ahead, toward the enemy. The Japanese crews were either incapacitated by the acrid fumes or possibly so shocked by the sight and smell that they were unable to return fire effectively. Very quickly the turtle boat crews fired their guns, savagely raking the sides of the enemy craft and causing great confusion and carnage among the Japanese.

After a series of decisive engagements Yi soundly won the day, inflicting such severe damage on the Japanese forces that they were forced to withdraw. So complete was the Korean victory that it would be more than three hundred years before the Japanese again attempted an invasion of Korea.

Admiral Yi died during the final battle, in circumstances identical to those that would later cause the death of Admiral Nelson at the Battle of Trafalgar—Yi refused to hear the pleas of his officers to seek shelter during the height of the battle and, like Nelson, fell victim to gunfire from an enemy vessel.

A Boat, a Plane, or What?

I think I can, I think I can, I think I can . . . FLY!
cried the little boat, as all the other boats in the marina laughed.

—J. GREGORY DILL

While the line above might have been taken from some twisted children's story about a little boat suffering a schizophrenic episode, it in fact describes a former Soviet engineering reality.

In the 1960s a US spy satellite photographed what appeared to be a large aircraft under construction near the city of Gorky, in what was then the Soviet Union. The CIA alerted the Pentagon and continued to monitor the building of this very large and curious craft, which would later be dubbed the Caspian Sea Monster.

Eventually it became obvious to the experts examining updated satellite images that what they were really viewing was not a conventional aircraft, but rather a hybrid boat-plane of a kind never before seen. What the Pentagon people were actually looking at was a full-sized working model of an *ekranoplan*, designed by comrade Rostislav Yevgenyvich Alekseev, a former ship designer, pilot, and auto racing aficionado. Rostislav Yevgenyvich was the quintessential Russian Tim Allen when it came to power and speed—more was always definitely better!

Alekseev, evidently an early advocate of extreme sports, gave his bureaucratic superiors ulcers with his dangerous high-speed driving habits and reckless downhill skiing. But he was also a creative genius who had moved far beyond the development of hydrofoil watercraft into a completely new area of research. He and his staff designed and built a three-hundred-foot craft, displacing five hundred metric tons, that could "fly" at a maximum of ten feet above the surface of the water at a speed of almost three hundred knots, with the assistance of a force known as ground effect. This phenomenon, well known to all aircraft pilots, occurs when an airfoil moves in close proximity to a ground or a water surface. The airfoil's lifting ability increases and drag decreases, causing a cushion of air to develop beneath the aircraft. By "flying" at an altitude of only ten feet, and staying in ground effect, Alekseev's "monster" had the military potential to move large numbers of troops and heavy weapons extremely quickly and economically (fuel-wise) at an altitude that would make detection by surface radar almost impossible.

Unfortunately for the brilliant and eccentric Alekseev, construction of further *ekranoplans* ceased with the end of the Cold War and the disintegration of the former Soviet Union. Now some of Alekseev's former associates hope to develop large passenger-carrying *ekranoplans* for commercial transport across large bodies of water.

A number of companies around the world are presently working on wing-in-ground effect (WIG) craft based on Alekseev's considerable research. By combining the economy of ship transport with the speed of aircraft, economical carriage of passengers and freight might be just around the corner. There may, however, be some unforeseen problems with such hybrids. Will the captain of such a craft be required to hold a master's ticket from the Coast Guard as well as a commercial pilot's license from the FAA? And what about the danger posed to sailors? A typical automated container ship bearing down on a cruising sailboat is bad enough. But what about an *ekranoplan* coming your way at almost three hundred knots, just ten feet above the water? Better stow a spare mast!

Roman Exploration of the New World?

Just as we were finally getting used to the idea that Leif Eriksson had established the first European settlement in America, at L'Anse aux Meadows in Newfoundland, long before Columbus set out on his voyage of exploration, we are left to wonder if even the tenacious Norsemen might have been beaten in their westward voyages of discovery by citizens of ancient Rome.

That remarkable idea now seems possible given the following discovery. Anthropologist Romeo H. Hristov has studied a small bust of a bearded Roman seaman discovered at a burial site some forty miles west of Mexico City. Hristov had samples of the bust material dated to about 200 CE, and experts identified the object as unquestionably of Roman origin. The head sports a hat resembling a knitted woolen cap called a *pylos* that was popular with Greek sailors. In fact, it looks surprisingly like a modern sailor's watch cap!

But is it possible ancient Romans could have sailed to America? By about 600 BCE, Phoenician sailors had explored most of the Mediterranean and had even made a coastal circumnavigation of the African continent. These voyages prompted Hanno, a fifth century BCE navigator from Carthage in North Africa, to sail through the Pillars of Hercules (Straits of Gibraltar) to explore southward along the Atlantic coast of Africa and to establish settlements as far south as Senegal. When the Romans, under consul Caius Duilius, destroyed the Carthaginian fleet in 260 BCE, it is quite possible they might have gained valuable knowledge from captured Carthaginian navigators concerning the greater world lying beyond Gibraltar.

It would not tax a modern sailor's mind too much to imagine a Roman vessel, its large square sail filled by northeast trade winds, cruising downwind to the north coast of South America. If only one literate captain had perused the works of Roman geographer Sebosus, the voyage would seem to be quite possible. Sebosus described the land of the

Hesperides, the "most westerly land of the world where the weather is always mild." Furthermore, Sebosus advised that Hesperides landfall could be made after only "forty days' sail" westward from the Cape Verde Islands, just off the coast of Senegal.

A typical Roman merchant ship of the time might have been a sturdy enough vessel for such a trip. The Roman *corbita* was a stoutly built craft, often as large as five hundred gross tons. With a brave, adventurous crew it might easily have made the downwind voyage from the Cape Verde Islands to the New World, making landfall on the Venezuelan coast of South America in the time suggested by Sebosus.

It is intriguing to imagine a Roman standard-bearer (seven to eight hundred years before Leif Eriksson's voyage to Newfoundland) trudging ashore behind his captain onto some South American beach to claim this new world for the Senate and people of Rome, then thrusting his staff, topped with Rome's Imperial Eagle and the letters SPQR, into a sandy beach. But maybe even the Romans were not the first to land in the New World. Pottery has been found at excavations in Ecuador that looks suspiciously like pottery made in Japan.

Eventually it may prove entirely possible that adventurous, sea-roving *Homo sapiens* have been rediscovering the Americas on a more or less regular basis over the last few thousand years.

Piracy

It is, it is a glorious thing
To be a Pirate King . . .

—*Pirates of Penzance* by Gilbert and Sullivan

These lines from the Gilbert and Sullivan operetta perpetuate the centuries-old myth of romantic ocean piracy. The image of a lusty bronzed Adonis, cutlass at hand, swinging back aboard his ship carrying a swooning, impossibly bosomed Venus has adorned the covers of adventure novels for at least fifty years. But the myth and the fact have little in common.

The word *pirate* first appeared about 140 BCE as the Latin *peirato*. But pirates seem to have been around for at least as long as sailors have been plowing the sea. In fact, piracy might just be the world's second oldest profession. Acts of piracy have been recorded in virtually every era, with clay tablets recording pirate raids on North African settlements during the reign of Pharaoh Ikhnaton twenty-three hundred years ago. Even Homer's *Odyssey* mentions piracy as a well-established marine activity.

The Roman era saw Mediterranean Sea commerce brought almost to a standstill by roving pirate vessels. In the years from about 800 to 1100 CE, the most notable European pirates were the Vikings, who plundered and pillaged as far east as the Baltic shores of Russia and as far south as North Africa. In Asia, as China's empire fell into decline during the thirteenth to sixteenth centuries, pirate fleets began raiding trading junks and coastal towns along the Yangtze River Delta. The fifteenth and sixteenth centuries also saw the rise of North African corsairs, who eventually attacked vessels as far afield as the coasts of Newfoundland and Iceland.

But it was the late seventeenth and early eighteenth centuries that saw the rise of the truly classic age of pirating portrayed in novels such as *Treasure Island.* During this time many future infamous figures began their careers as law-abiding mariners who obtained commissions or letters of marque from their respective monarchs to harass enemy ships during times of war. When the wars ended, many of these licensed pirates (privateers) found it difficult to give up the easy money, and so fell into true piracy, taking any vessel that sailed across their course. (See chapter 1 for an explanation of the terms *letters of marque* and *privateer.*) The notorious Edward (Blackbeard) Teach became the terror of the coasts of the Carolinas, while female pirates Mary Read and Anne Bonny raided Spanish, Dutch, and British vessels in the Caribbean with their shared lover, "Handsome Jack" Rackham.

Today there are still reports of piracy and pirate activity, especially attacks on cargo ships in the Far East by gangs of well-armed bandits in high-speed boats. Interested readers might wish to browse either the International Chamber of Commerce Commercial Crime Services (ICC-CCS) Web site (www.icc-ccs.org/prc/piracyreport.php) to read recent commercial piracy reports or Noonsite Limited's Web site (www.noonsite.com/General/Piracy), which also includes useful information and recent reports of pirate activity.

With pirate attacks still occurring on both private and large commercial vessels in some parts of the world, a visit to the above-mentioned sites might be a good idea for those planning offshore cruising. Any visit by pirates will likely not be as entertaining or amusing as those celebrated in Gilbert and Sullivan's memorable lyrics.

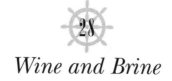

Wine and Brine

When divers from the Netherlands Institute for Ship and Underwater Archeology were investigating the wreck of an unidentified Dutch warship off the north coast of Holland a few years ago, they could not have imagined finding an intact, three-century-old bottle of wine amid the marine detritus on the ocean floor.

European wine commentators and connoisseurs were in a perfect frenzy when news of the three-hundred-year-old find was announced. When the heavy green glass bottle was finally uncorked, a special panel of wine experts agreed that the contents tasted surprisingly good, considering the wine's unconventional mode of storage—under the sea. But they did whine a bit about its unpleasant "nose," which apparently was reminiscent of the sulfide stench a sailor might encounter downwind of a South American oil refinery, at low tide.

Wine has been around for at least ten millennia and has been going to sea with mariners, as both victual and cargo, for at least the last four thousand years. In fact, Genesis 9 reports that the first thing celebrated yachtsman and zoologist Noah did after running the Ark aground on Mount Ararat was to set about planting a vineyard. By the time the ancient Greeks were setting courses for southern Italy, wine was a staple beverage at sea. On a voyage wine would keep considerably better than water, which after only a few weeks would be host to all sorts of disagreeable flora and fauna. A happy circumstance since any sailor would have preferred wine over water anyway, even if his ship's water supply was unspoiled.

In Roman times wine was one of the most widely traded commodities in the Mediterranean. Cargo vessels laden with wine amphorae—large, tapered two-handled clay jars with narrow necks, sealed with cork and covered over with a sealer to protect the nearly seven gallons of wine each held—sailed as far as the remote island Britannia (modern Britain) to supply expatriate Romans with a little taste of home, and civilization.

Shipping wine by sea was quite economical. It cost about the same to ship one amphora the entire length of the Mediterranean as it did to transport the same amphora one hundred miles on land. It was for this reason that most early vineyards were deliberately situated near coastlines with good access to the sea.

When vineyards on the island of Madeira began producing and exporting wines for markets as far away as India and Japan, shippers began to notice a very interesting phenomenon. It was common practice at the time to return all unsold wine from these distant markets to the port of Funchal at Madeira. When these "traveled" wines were returned and finally opened and tasted, their flavor was found to be much superior to the "untraveled" wines in storage. Somehow the hot temperatures of the equator and the rough passage around the Cape of Good Hope—twice—worked some magic on the precious contents of the barrels stowed deep in the holds of cargo ships.

Perhaps that unfortunate Dutch captain of three centuries ago was simply carrying his store of wine on board in hopes its quality would improve by abusing it a bit at sea. Little could he have suspected that his carefully stowed wine would become the center of such scrutiny, almost three hundred years after his ship slipped beneath the waves.

29

America

Whﬤen New York Yacht Club Commodore John Stevens ordered the building of the schooner yacht *America*, he could hardly have imagined the remarkable career his dream racer would have.

In 1851 Stevens asked designer George Steers for a racing schooner of about 170 tons that could win a sixty-mile race around the Isle of Wight in Great Britain. Steers designed a very clean two-masted schooner with a length of 94 feet, beam of 22.5 feet, and draft of 11.5 feet.

The stoical old salts of the Royal Yacht Squadron must have needed extra starch for those famous stiff upper lips while they watched painfully as Stevens's "colonial upstart" schooner, the only American entry, sailed to a first-place victory ahead of fourteen of Britain's finest and fastest yachts. Even worse, a young Queen Victoria witnessed the humiliating finish. When the queen asked who was in second place, a dismayed attendant lamented, "Your Majesty, there is no second."

The cup presented to the victorious American crew became the America's Cup in honor of the little schooner's name. But the yacht *America* was destined to have even more interesting sailing adventures.

America remained in Britain for seven years after her stunning victory, until she was purchased by Lord Templeton and renamed *Camilla*. When the American Civil War began, *Camilla* was back across the Atlantic at the port of Savannah, Georgia. Templeton, seeing a chance to make a buck (or rather a quid), sold her to the Confederate government, which quickly fitted her out with deck guns, in preparation for employing the speedy little racer as a blockade-runner. It was during her final blockade run for the South that she was pursued by vessels of the blockading US fleet up into the St. Johns River in Florida, where she became trapped. Her desperate crew, fearing she would be captured and used against the Confederacy, quickly scuttled her.

Enterprising Federal forces, ironically led by a another Stevens—Lieutenant Thomas Stevens—successfully raised *Camilla* and commissioned her into the US Navy, where she carried out a number of naval duties and participated in the blockade of Charleston Harbor. But in 1863 she was relieved of war duty, renamed *America*, and sailed to Newport, Rhode Island, to become a training vessel for the US Naval Academy.

In 1870 *America* was relieved of her teaching position at the Naval Academy to once again cross the Atlantic, as a defender in the first America's Cup race. She finished a very respectable fourth among the twenty-three defenders and beat the British challenger, *Cambria*, by thirteen minutes.

Benjamin Butler bought *America* in 1873 to use as a personal cruising and racing yacht, and as late as 1901 she was still racing. But a long period of decline for the schooner soon followed. Her keel was scavenged for lead to make bullets for the US Army sent to Europe during World War I. By 1921 *America*'s glory days were definitely over. She was riddled with rotten timber, and no one seemed to want her. *America* was presented to Marblehead's Eastern Yacht Club, which in turn sent her back to the Naval Academy for preservation.

America ended her career in circumstances as strange as her eclectic life. In 1942 she was crushed beyond repair when the roof of the building in which she was stored collapsed under the weight of wet snow. After a life spanning almost a hundred years, the famous yacht that had brought such prestige to American yacht racing was reduced to little more than firewood.

30

The Stone Fleet

Anyone familiar with that old sailor's last lament, "The Stone Fleet" by Herman (*Moby Dick*) Melville, will recall that the intentionally doomed fleet celebrated in his poem was composed mostly of old whaling vessels collected from the ports of Fairhaven and New Bedford.

The idea for the stone fleet was conceived during the early days of the Civil War, when it was decided that Union forces should set up and maintain a blockade of Southern ports and waterways to stem the flow of munitions and supplies to the Confederacy. The blockade was also supposed to prevent Southern cash crops such as cotton from reaching world markets, thus depriving the Jefferson Davis government of badly needed foreign currency. The first part of the plan included Union patrol of entrances to major Southern ports like Charleston, South Carolina. The second and more radical approach was to sink navigational obstructions in enemy harbors and channels. It was at this point the plan for the stone fleet was put forward.

At a July 1861 meeting in Washington, a supremely confident Gustavus Fox, assistant secretary of the navy, fidgeted while waiting to float a sinking idea. His brilliant concept: Collect old sailing vessels, overballast them with rock debris, sail them into Confederate waters, and then sink them at the most effective points to block enemy and neutral shipping to all but the smallest of vessels. Fox suggested most of the vessels needed could be found tied up and idle at various whaling ports in New England.

When the Civil War had begun in 1861, the New England whaling industry was already in a decline. Petroleum had been discovered in Pennsylvania in 1859, giving America kerosene, a cheap replacement for the whale oil then used in lamps. Also, the development of inexpensive spring steel had lessened the need for whalebone in the construction of women's corsets. If that wasn't bad enough, whale numbers were declining, necessitating longer and more expensive voyages.

Fox's scheme was eagerly adopted and, by November 1861, US Navy agents were buying all the old ships they could find—paying ten dollars per ton. They also bought granite with which to sink them. Owners of whaling ships eagerly sold their rotting vessels to recover some of their investment. Holes were bored in the vessels' bottoms, then securely plugged, and the granite was loaded aboard for the voyage south. When the ships arrived at the designated points, they would be positioned and the plugs knocked out to sink them.

The first stone fleet was sunk at the entrance to Charleston Harbor on December 20, 1861. But Confederate blockade-runners quickly found that they could easily and safely slip through a passage called Mafitts Channel to reach the sea. For that reason Fox decided to sink a second stone fleet to close that channel also. The sinking of these vessels caused great consternation in European capitals and resulted in many shipping nations complaining bitterly to Washington that such actions were both "barbarous and an outrage to civilized Christian nations."

The Europeans, however, needn't have bothered. The sly old Fox's stone fleet idea flopped. The heavy granite ballast pushed the scuttled ships deep into the soft ooze of the bottom, where the wooden, worm-eaten hulls quickly broke up. In fact, the sinkings had the opposite effect from their intended purpose—navigation in Charleston Harbor was actually substantially improved by the sinkings. Scuttling the ships resulted in narrowing the harbor's mouth, which caused the speed of the water to increase in several places. This eroded bottom sediments, effectively deepening the channels.

The utter failure of the plan—which sacrificed a significant portion of New England's whaling heritage—led Melville to end his poem somewhat bitterly with the following lines:

> *And all for naught. The waters pass . . .*
> *Currents will have their way;*
> *Nature is nobody's ally; 'tis well;*
> *The Harbor is bettered . . . will stay.*
> *A failure, and complete,*
> *Was your Old Stone Fleet.*

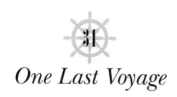

One Last Voyage

In the opening year of World War I the German naval cruiser SMS *Emden* and her crew found themselves in the South Pacific, charged with upholding the imperial interests of Germany's Kaiser William. On November 9, 1914, at 6:30 AM, the commander of *Emden* ordered Kapitanleutnant Helmuth Karl von Mucke and fifty men ashore at Direction Island, in the Keeling island group, to destroy the vital enemy cable and radio station located on the lonely outpost.

The landing party quickly vandalized the facility and the British operators of the station were officially told they were prisoners, although no one was actually constrained or locked up. In fact, the interaction of the Germans and the British was so cordial that Von Mucke agreed to a desperate British request that the station's radio tower be toppled in such a manner as to avoid ruining the tennis court adjacent to the station—tennis being the only real diversion the British had to combat the boredom born of remote island existence.

Unknown to the landing party, as they set about their selectively destructive chores, an Australian naval cruiser was patrolling in the neighborhood. By pure chance, HMAS *Sydney* received and responded to an emergency distress message sent by the British radio operator on duty as the Germans arrived. *Sydney* discovered *Emden* offshore and immediately gave chase, followed by a spirited two-hour running gun battle. By the time the German shore party returned to the rendezvous point to meet their ship, they discovered *Emden* nowhere in sight. The Australian cruiser and *Emden* fought a wide-ranging, pitched battle, but in the end *Sydney* was victorious and *Emden* was destroyed.

When the German shore party eventually discovered what had happened to their ship, and with possible capture by an armed shore party from *Sydney* imminent, Von Mucke decided to commandeer a rotting sailing vessel he discovered lying at anchor near the destroyed radio station. The three-masted *Ayesha*, square-rigged on her foremast and fore- and aft-rigged on her main and mizzen, was owned by the Clunies-Ross family and had originally been used in the copra trade between Direction Island and Batavia. Von Mucke, having gained experience on sailing vessels before entering the naval service, immediately recognized the ship for what she was, an old hulk well past her "best before" date. But even though her condition would have made any marine surveyor cringe, the German officer quickly decided to ready the tired old ship for sea in a desperate bid to make a run for home and avoid capture by the enemy.

Some of Von Mucke's men had also had sail training experience, while others were former fishermen. So, while their less sail-wise comrades scouted the island for provisions, those who had spent some time before the mast set about bringing mildewed canvas topside from *Ayesha*'s sail locker and replacing some of the worst of the rotted rigging. Von Mucke went below to gingerly poke about at *Ayesha*'s spongy timbers, looking for structural problems. Eventually he stopped probing—every part of the ship was structurally unsound.

The British, apparently wishing not to appear poor sports even during wartime, watched the German preparations closely. In a surprising show of gratitude for the sparing of their beloved tennis court, the station's men actively assisted the Germans in locating provisions. They also helped prepare *Ayesha* for sea, and even congregated on the beach to cheer the Germans off as they departed on what most thought a brave but foolhardy voyage back to *der Vaterland*.

The ancient sailing vessel was soon at sea on a northeast course for the island of Sumatra, but with her home island hardly out of sight and in a freshening breeze, *Ayesha*'s rotten shrouds began snapping like taut violin strings. The crew were soon constantly employed with unending repairs to both rigging and sails. To make matters worse, a British cruiser like *Sydney* might be expected to appear at any moment. The concussion from enemy guns alone would probably reduce the sickly ship to so much floating debris, even if no shells actually hit her.

Von Mucke decided to shape a course for the port of Padang on Sumatra. He felt chances were good that *Ayesha* might be allowed to enter Padang, a neutral port under Dutch control, to make more extensive repairs. Before arriving off the port in late November, Von Mucke ordered his men to cut four gun ports in *Ayesha* to accommodate the four machine guns the landing party had taken on their Direction Island raid. This move, he decided, would convince Dutch authorities that "SMS" *Ayesha* was, indeed, an armed German man-of-war. As such, she could not be interned as a merchant vessel would be upon entering a neutral port during wartime. On arrival, the Dutch authorities reluctantly accepted his arguments, but insisted *Ayesha* be out of their jurisdiction before nightfall to avoid diplomatic problems with the British.

The short stay in port did not allow time for substantial repairs, but several German merchant vessels already interned in the port managed to send over their ships' boats filled with books, clothes, cigarettes, and outdated German newspapers—significantly lifting the morale of *Ayesha*'s crew. Through the German consul in the port they also received charts, spare canvas for sail repair, fresh water, personal items such as razors for the crew, and even some live pigs for later slaughter to provide fresh meat. At eight bells *Ayesha* shipped her anchor with some difficulty before again getting under way.

On December 14, while *Ayesha* was lying to in heavy seas and rain, a lookout called from the tops to report an approaching vessel. At first Von Mucke believed the intruder to be an Australian or British cruiser about to pounce on his ailing *Ayesha*. He was greatly relieved to find the mystery ship was the steamer *Choising*, a German vessel. *Choising*'s captain had received news of *Ayesha*'s improbable voyage by radio from Padang and had immediately begun searching for her. The following morning, after the storm had blown itself out, *Ayesha* lay dead in the water. The steamer took the old ship in tow, but Von Mucke finally decided he and his crew should remain aboard *Choising*. He ordered his men to scuttle *Ayesha*.

Von Mucke and his crew finally prepared to bid farewell to their commandeered ship. *Ayesha* had reached the end of her long sailing career after a final voyage of seventeen hundred nautical miles through storm- and enemy-patrolled waters. As he and his crew looked on, *Ayesha* slipped graciously beneath the waves off the southern Maldives—a far more dignified end for the old workhorse than a slow death, rotting away at anchor.

The fate of the pigs is unknown, but it seems likely they perished as a result of consumption.

32

Boxer *Knocked Out*

The state of Maine has always been an angler's and hunter's paradise, even during the War of 1812. Between June and August His Majesty's Brig *Boxer*, thirty-year-old Lieutenant Samuel Blyth commanding, found the coastal "fishing" particularly rewarding. In that short space of time, and with little effort, she had captured the unarmed American schooners *Rebecca, Fortune, Fairplay, Two Brothers,* and the sloop *Friendship* as prizes.

Only a few weeks earlier Blyth had been a member of the funeral cortege for American Captain James Lawrence at Halifax, following Lawrence's death aboard the US Frigate *Chesapeake* (see chapter 5). The exceptional good luck the Royal Navy vessel enjoyed made Blyth decide to anchor inside Penguin Point, a short distance from Monhegan Island on the hostile Maine coast, to give his crew a little well-deserved rest and relaxation.

Boxer's surgeon, the captain of the Royal Marines assigned to the ship, and two midshipmen decided to indulge themselves in a bit of sport by rowing ashore for a little pigeon shooting, while the remainder of the small crew and the captain stayed aboard the brig. As the morning wore on some of the crew found comfortable areas on deck to read or grab a few hours' sleep, while others took advantage of the rest period to repair clothing or play cards. But the peace of the forenoon was soon broken when *Boxer*'s masthead lookout spied a sail creeping over the eastern horizon. Very quickly the lookout identified the sail as belonging to another armed brig. In minutes *Boxer* was standing to sea, leaving the four surprised pigeon hunters stranded on shore.

The sail belonged to the US Brig *Enterprise*, Lieutenant William Burrows commanding. Like Blyth, Burrows was young—only twenty-eight years old. His orders were to seek out and destroy all New Brunswick and Nova Scotia privateers found preying upon New England mercantile shipping. *Enterprise* was slightly larger than *Boxer*, but her main advantage lay in her having a full complement of men aboard. *Boxer*, as well as being short her surgeon, captain of marines, and two midshipmen, had also earlier dispatched a large portion of her crew to sail captured prizes to the ports of Saint John and Halifax.

By noon the two brigs had closed the distance between them to fewer than five miles, and their crews had been beaten to quarters to prepare for action. But the capricious winds of coastal Maine died without warning, leaving the two vessels some four miles apart for a time, trapped in a flat calm. When the wind again sprang up from the southwest, each commander attempted to maneuver his brig to best advantage, upwind of his enemy. In the end it was Burrows's *Enterprise* that gained the weather gauge, and by three o'clock both brigs were on a starboard tack with *Enterprise* windward of *Boxer*. When less than a pistol shot apart, both *Enterprise* and *Boxer* fired full broadsides simultaneously in a deafening, fiery roar.

The damage to both brigs became obvious as smoke from the first broadsides drifted away. The carnage was horrific! The gun crews of both brigs worked frantically, slipping on decks now slick with blood and gore, to reload. Both commanders had been hit in the opening exchange of fire, Blyth dying instantly, shot having ripped away his arm and shoulder. Burrows, too, was hit and mortally wounded by bar shot from *Boxer*'s guns. Although slowly bleeding to death, Burrows remained conscious for a time, issuing orders and refusing to be taken below. For fifteen minutes a weltering exchange of gunfire continued. On *Boxer*'s deck Lieutenant McCreery assumed his fallen captain's place, while on *Enterprise* Lieutenant McColl relieved the dying Burrows.

By four o'clock the Royal Navy's *Boxer* was the clear loser and her crew had had enough. Because most of her lines had been damaged and her ensign could not be lowered to announce her surrender, Blyth's linen dining room tablecloth was hastily nailed up on *Boxer*'s mainmast as a signal to *Enterprise* of her capitulation. Lieutenant Burrows of *Enterprise* lived just long enough to receive his worldly reward for his ship's battle success—the presentation of Captain Blyth's sword.

Unknown to the combatants, a sailor had climbed the observatory tower at Portland's Munjoy Hill to observe the battle through the powerful French-built telescope installed there to spot vessels inbound for Portland Harbor. From this high perspective, the seaman called out a blow-by-blow description of the battle to a group of interested Portland citizens gathered below the tower, as an announcer might cover a sporting event today.

With the battle over, the battered but victorious *Enterprise* set a course for Portland, followed in her wake by the even more battered and badly beaten *Boxer*. In a truly ironic twist, the bodies of Captain Blyth and Lieutenant Burrows were buried with full military honors in side-by-side graves at Portland's Eastern Cemetery. Every Memorial Day each grave is decorated with a national flag, Burrows's with the Stars and Stripes and Blyth's with a Union Jack.

There is no record of how many pigeons *Boxer*'s shooting party bagged, but evidently there was sufficient meat to sustain the four men during their long walk up the Bay of Fundy coast to the British town of Saint John, New Brunswick.

33

Seaman and Samurai

In the history of ocean navigation and exploration, names such as Leif Eriksson, Ferdinand Magellan, and Vasco da Gama shine as brightly as Venus on a clear night at sea. But what of those lesser-known European-born navigators who have not made the "first string" on the pages of navigational history?

One of those second-stringers was William Adams, an English navigator born at Kent, England, in 1564, the same year as William Shakespeare. Young Will apprenticed at a London shipyard, learning shipbuilding skills by day and studying navigation at night. By the time he was twenty-five he was already an experienced navigator, having served with Sir Francis Drake's victorious Armada-routing navy.

Adams evidently tired of life in England, possibly sensing that more interesting adventures awaited him beyond far distant seas. At a time when other English seamen were looking to make their fortunes by sailing west to the lucrative Newfoundland fishery, Adams chose to seek his fortune by shaping a course to the Far East.

With résumé in hand Adams bade his wife, children, and England adieu to set off for Holland, where his credentials would earn him a position as pilot major (chief navigator). In 1598 he sailed in a five-ship convoy for the East Indies via the Straits of Magellan. As fate would have it, Adams's ship was the only vessel of the original five to survive the voyage. Eventually, with a crew sick with scurvy but guided by Adams's competent navigation, the Dutch ship made landfall at the Japanese island of Kyushu in 1600.

Adams was possibly the first Englishman, although certainly not the first European, to reach the Land of the Rising Sun. Portuguese traders were already established there, and they feared that Adams's presence might jeopardize their lucrative trade monopoly. The Portuguese convinced the local warlord, Shogun Tokugawa Ieyasu, to imprison Adams and his Dutch shipmates, telling him these strangers would pose a serious threat to his regime.

Ieyasu met and questioned Adams many times while he was in prison, each time becoming more intrigued with the Englishman's intelligence and store of nautical knowledge. These meetings eventually led to a firm friendship, with the result that Adams and his men were finally released from detention. Adams began to teach Ieyasu the rudiments of geometry and navigation. Eventually the shogun asked Adams to instruct his shipwrights in the latest Western shipbuilding techniques. In response, Adams designed and oversaw the construction of an eighty-ton ship with which his Japanese host was very pleased—so much so that Ieyasu granted the navigator a twelve-ducat-per-year retainer (about twenty-eight dollars today) to act as his adviser.

As time passed, Adams became homesick for his family and England. Ieyasu, shrewd enough to recognize Adams for the valuable political and military asset the Englishman had become, flatly refused to allow him to return to England. But in a brilliant move, Ieyasu issued a decree that the Englishman Adams was now officially "dead." Ieyasu then bestowed a new name on Adams, Miura Anjin, and granted him the rank of samurai. Ieyasu also arranged for Adams to marry a girl named Oyuki, the beautiful daughter of one of the shogun's senior bureaucrats. To ensure that the door of the Englishman's "prison" was fully bolted, Ieyasu gave the newlyweds an impressive country estate that would provide Adams with a more lavish lifestyle than he could ever have hoped to achieve back in England.

In the years that followed, Adams fathered a son and daughter by Oyuki and supervised the building of a fleet of Western-style vessels for his master. He also became Ieyasu's trusted adviser on all matters pertaining to diplomacy and foreign trade. Ironically, Adams's influence became so great that even his old Portuguese enemies found they had to solicit his assistance to gain an audience with Ieyasu.

Adams died near Nagasaki in 1620, after years of loyal service to his Japanese lord, but without ever having made a return visit to England.

Aural Amputation Aggravates War

It's unlikely that former Secretary of State Dean Rusk had Captain Robert Jenkins in mind when he said: "One of the best ways to persuade others is with your ears." But that pearl of wisdom does seem rather apt, especially after learning about the infamous eighteenth-century English sailor.

In 1731 Captain Jenkins was master of the merchant brig *Rebecca*, navigating Caribbean waters and engaging in trade at various West Indian ports. One morning, while sailing off Havana Harbor, *Rebecca* was overhauled and boarded by Cuban Guarda Costa searching for contraband. The Spanish officer in charge of the boarding party evidently had some reason to suspect the Englishman's motives and may actually have found evidence aboard *Rebecca* that suggested Jenkins was engaged in smuggling—a charge Jenkins later vehemently denied back in England. Jenkins's account of the event said the Spanish boarders seized and off-loaded *Rebecca*'s cargo. Then, according to Jenkins, he was tortured and had one of his ears cut off. After a short period the English captain was released by the Spanish authorities and set adrift in *Rebecca*.

When the aurally challenged Jenkins finally arrived back in England, he complained bitterly to the government and press about his alleged torture at the hands of the Spanish, but his story initially fell on deaf ears. Jenkins did become a minor celebrity on the London pub circuit for a short time, though. Fellow seamen who were anxious to get a firsthand report, while having a pint, would invariably inquire of the unhappy captain, ". . . 'ere, Cap'n Jenkins, sor, tell us yer tale." Then for the next couple of hours Jenkins's listeners would be treated to an embellished yarn that was guaranteed to earn for him a bottomless tankard of ale. Of course, some pub patrons discounted at least part of his story, having heard that the captain's missing ear had in fact been chewed off during a drunken waterfront brawl in Jamaica by that rarest of creatures—an eighteenth-century sailor with enough teeth remaining to accomplish

the deed. Eventually, though, Captain Jenkins and his story began to re-
cede from the public consciousness.

Some seven years after the alleged aural amputation, however, relations between Britain and her perennial nemesis Spain had reached a
particularly low ebb. Anti-Spanish sentiments were running high among
Britain's wealthy merchant class after Spain had begun excluding English ships from lucrative trade with her colonies in the New World. Some
recalled Jenkins's tale from years earlier, and because both would now
prove useful in swaying public opinion, the story and Captain Jenkins
were promptly resurrected. Suddenly Jenkins's ear seemed to be on
every politician's lips. Propaganda spin doctors skillfully guided the tailor-
made story to an appropriate level of atrocity to nurture public outrage
and hatred of Spain, and at the same time (not coincidentally) promote
England's political and economic aspirations in the West Indies. Captain Jenkins's finest hour was at hand.

In 1738 Jenkins was summoned to appear before the House of Com-
mons to testify about his ordeal while in the hands of the Spanish.
Elated at the prospect, he spoke long and eloquently before the august
body, having by this time honed and fine-tuned the elements of his story
to near theatrical perfection. He so bedazzled those present with his or-
atorical contortions that he might have expected to receive for his reward several barrels of London's finest ale for this, his crowning
performance. When he reached the culmination of his well-rehearsed
epic, he played his trump card—dramatically removing from his waist-
coat pocket and waving high above his head the fabled and much publi-
cized ear, in all its shriveled glory. A collective parliamentary gasp
resounded through the House as all eyes fell upon that ear. The effect was
electric—the nation demanded that the severed relic be avenged, and that
the Iberian devils be made to pay. Indignation became so great that Prime
Minister Walpole was soon pressured into declaring war with Spain—a conflict that history would record as the "War of Jenkins' Ear" (1739–41).

However, despite all the righteous rhetoric and posturing in England, that country and Spain chose to wage the war with little or no enthusiasm. The conflict highlights consisted of a few minor sea skirmishes
in various parts of the Caribbean and an unsuccessful land attack by
Georgia's colonial Governor James Oglethorpe and his American forces
upon the Spanish garrison stationed in St. Augustine, Florida.

The war did, however, allow Captain Jenkins to bask in the national spotlight and enjoy his "fifteen minutes of fame." And just like any present-day celebrity, Jenkins cashed in on his newfound notoriety by writing a book about his Caribbean cruising experiences, published under the catchy title *Spanish Insolence Corrected by English Bravery*.

Despite some moderate success as a first-time author, Jenkins (evidently through his remaining intact ear) eventually heard the sea's call to take up his former nautical profession. In 1740 he accepted command of a British East India Company ship bound for the Far East. No doubt his choosing to sail in waters other than those of the Caribbean had less to do with seeking new horizons and more to do with being unwilling to risk shaping a course back to the West Indies where his remaining ear, or possibly some other valued part of his anatomy, might have been at risk of loss to a vengeful Spanish sword.

35

A Prince of a Navigator

Henry the Navigator was truly a prince among sailors in pre-Columbian Europe. Henry was born in 1394, the third son of King John of Portugal and his English bride, Queen Phillippa of the English House of Lancaster. Of the three sons, only Henry showed an early interest in promoting the arts of seafaring and navigation.

In 1420, while Henry was still a young man, his father appointed him governor of Portugal's Algarve coast. His first act was to construct a naval observatory at Sagres near Cape St. Vincent in southern Portugal for the study of astronomy. Later he established a school of seamanship and navigation at the same location. Henry eventually coaxed many of the foremost scientific minds from the Middle East and Europe to live and work at Sagres. The academic compound became a fifteenth-century nautical "think tank" where the very keenest intellects met to unravel the mysteries of the celestial sphere, study navigation, and refine and further develop the crude magnetic compass then in use.

As the fifteenth century unfolded, little was known of the world beyond the boundaries of the European continent. Seamen rarely sailed out of the sight of land or deviated from established trading routes for fear of encountering sea monsters or sirens, or possibly falling off the edge of the earth. By 1425 the growing eclectic academic community at Sagres boasted Arab mathematicians and mapmakers, Jewish astronomers and translators, Spanish geographers fleeing the Inquisition, experienced Norse seafarers, as well as pilots from the ports of Venice and Genoa—the community embraced anyone whose skills could further the understanding and exploration of the world's oceans and navigation upon them.

At Henry's order, yards in the nearby port of Lagos were outfitted for shipbuilding and staffed with all those whose skills were required—carpenters, shipwrights, smiths, sail makers, coopers, rope makers, victualers, and the most experienced seamen. Back in Sagres, specialists labored to develop more seaworthy designs for vessels, increasing both hull strength and size to accommodate longer voyages, and ultimately developing innovative new ship designs like the caravel that would be built at the Lagos yards.

Soon Henry began to organize and equip sailing expeditions of discovery. The Azores and Madeira islands were rediscovered with his assistance, leading to their colonization. He instructed his captains to explore along the West African coast, but none would venture beyond dreaded Cape Bojador south of the Canary Islands because they feared the unknown (not an enviable trait for an ocean explorer).

Finally, in 1434, an expedition commander named Gil Eannes, on his second attempt, rounded the fearsome cape. Later expeditions, at great expense to Henry's treasury, sailed farther south, with Dinis Diaz rounding Cape Verde in 1445. These voyages marked the beginning of the age of European trade in black African slaves. Each successive expedition brought back more and more slaves to Portugal, resulting in ever-increasing profits for the country.

Henry died in 1460, thirty-two years before Columbus was to make his famous voyage. The improved compass and the caravel ship design that Henry had promoted contributed much to the navigational success of Columbus's first voyage.

Ironically, the man known as Henry the Navigator never actually sailed on any of the many voyages of discovery that he had sponsored.

36

Spying on the Weather

When Commander Peter Schrewe of freshly minted German *U-boat 537* ordered his vessel's lines cast off at the port of Kiel in the early-morning hours of September 18, 1943, both he and his youthful crew were still in the dark concerning their first mission.

The crew had arrived back at their new boat after shore leave to find strange metal canisters stowed where there should have been torpedoes for use in attacking Allied shipping. And there were two mysterious passengers aboard, too—an almost unheard-of occurrence on a U-boat on wartime patrol, except for the occasional reporter or spy catching a ride to a foreign shore. But the senior passenger didn't look much like a newspaperman, or a spy for that matter. Instead, the older civilian had the manner of a genial professor whom one might expect to find in a Stuttgart University lecture hall. The strangers were scientist Dr. Kurt Sommermeyer and his technical assistant.

After reaching the open Atlantic, Schrewe opened his sealed orders, read them, and announced *U-537*'s mission to the crew. Schrewe's instructions were to avoid contact with enemy vessels and, instead, set a course for the northern coast of Labrador to erect an automated weather recording and transmitting station on North American soil.

Knowing what the weather was like in the waters around Newfoundland has always been an essential bit of intelligence for any prudent navigator of the North Atlantic. But the Germans particularly needed timely and accurate weather data to assist them in more effectively directing their aggressive U-boat operations and predicting with some accuracy the timing and routes likely to be taken by outbound Halifax and New York convoys attempting to avoid the worst of North Atlantic weather. Siemens Company designed the automated station carried aboard *U-537*, which was designated WFL 26 or *Wetterfungerat-Land 26* (Automated Land Weather Station 26). WFL 26 was code-named Kurt for the Siemens employee who was responsible for the station's assembly in Labrador.

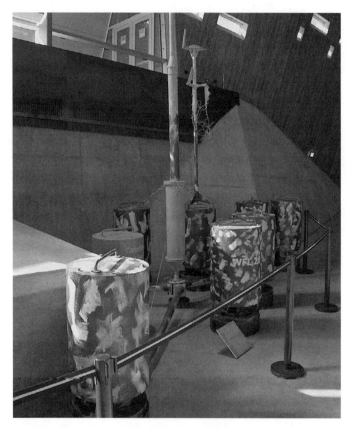

These weather station components were delivered to the coast of Labrador in 1943 and assembled into an automated weather station by Dr. Kurt Sommermeyer and the crew of U-boat 537.
J. Gregory Dill, courtesy Canadian War Museum, Ottawa, Canada

U-537's journey toward Labrador was fraught with dangers not only from Allied air and sea forces, but also from the turbulent Atlantic itself. At one point the sub was forced to surface in hurricane conditions to recharge batteries, an action that resulted in her large anti-aircraft gun being ripped from her hull by mountainous seas.

The submarine entered Martin Bay, Labrador, on October 22, and under Dr. Sommermeyer's direction the canisters and masts making up WFL 26 were carefully manhandled to the deck. Each of the canisters weighed approximately 220 pounds, making for awkward transport in rubber dinghies across the choppy water of the bay to the shore—a difficult "shingle" beach. Once landed, the station components had to be muscled up to a small plateau 170 feet above the water. There Dr. Sommermeyer directed the assembly of the prefabricated weather station components. One of the canisters, deliberately labeled in English to appear as if the station had been erected by Canadian authorities, was a ruse meant to satisfy the curiosity of anyone who might happen upon the isolated installation.

WFL 26 consisted of measurement modules for wind speed, direction, temperature, and barometric pressure, as well as advanced and massive, long-life nickel-cadmium batteries to power a 150-watt radio transmitter for broadcasting all collected data to German weather forecasters. The system was ingeniously designed so that the heavy batteries acted as anchors for the Lorenz-designed radio and instrument masts, securing them during high winds. A cylinder with conducting pins in one module formed Morse code letters when it rotated to identify the station to German receivers and also identify each measurement character. The radio transmitter was set to broadcast on a frequency of 3.94 megahertz at intervals during the day. To save battery power the design required the transmitter to be on for only three minutes during each reporting broadcast.

Finally, after successfully testing the operation of the automatic station, and after thirty tense hours having his vessel lying exposed on the surface in enemy waters, Commander Schrewe got *U-537* under way on a course for the south coast of Newfoundland.

Ironically, *U-537* met her end a year later on November 9, 1944, while on a Far East patrol. She was attacked and sunk with all hands by the submarine USS *Flounder,* almost halfway around the world from where she had delivered the Third Reich's only automated North American weather station. Dr. Sommermeyer, his assistant, and one of the crew survived the war. The crew member, Werner Bendler, left *U-537* when it returned to base. By a stroke of good luck, he was sent for officer training and so missed *U-537*'s doomed voyage to the Pacific.

In a final irony, WFL 26 managed only a few transmissions before an operational glitch silenced it forever, only days after its assembly. Incredibly, WFL 26 remained a well-kept secret for almost thirty-seven years. In the summer of 1980, the crew of a Canadian Coast Guard ship discovered Dr. Sommermeyer's automated weather station. The rusted remnants have been stabilized, authentically repainted, and put on display at the new Canadian War Museum in Ottawa.

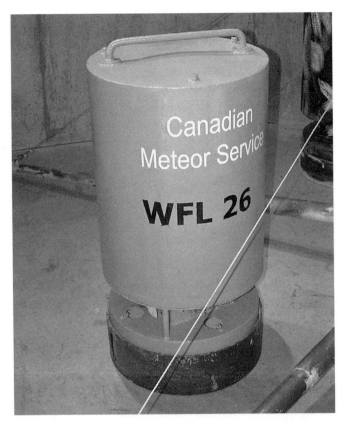

This weather station component was lettered to suggest the station was set up by Canadian weather services, a ruse to satisfy anyone who might find it. J. Gregory Dill, courtesy Canadian War Museum, Ottawa, Canada

The display of the German weather station stands as testament to a remote weather technology that eventually was refined and employed to contribute to the safety and peace of mind of seamen—the reverse of WFL 26's original deployment purpose, which was to assist in the destruction of Allied mariners and their ships.

POSTSCRIPT

I am indebted to John Corneil, head of collection information at the Canadian War Museum, and volunteer Bruno Friesen for research assistance for this story.

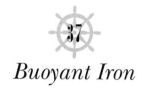

Buoyant Iron

The Industrial Revolution fed on a diet of coal, but grew on a framework of iron. It was inevitable, then, that innovative men of the period would seek creative new uses for the strong, versatile metal.

John Wilkinson of Britain was the undisputed king of the iron industry in the eighteenth century. Brilliant and eccentric, Wilkinson envisioned a world made of iron and became wealthy by creating new markets for the metal that included constructing what was probably the world's first vessel with an iron hull—a river barge built two years before the French Revolution.

Although Wilkinson's barge demonstrated conclusively to the skeptical that an iron-built hull would actually float, shipyards in Britain did not immediately rush to experiment with the novel idea of constructing ships of iron. In fact, it was not until the 1830s that iron-hulled sailing and steam vessels began to appear in any number.

Of iron-built vessels, *Nautical Magazine* enthusiastically reported in 1834:

> The importance of these vessels is daily increasing in general estimation, arising from the peculiar advantages they possess, of being not only water-tight and very durable, but, from their cleanliness, peculiarly healthy and desirable vessels. They afford no harbour for vermin, like those of wood, and in warm climates, the great conducting power of the metal gives off the heat to the water, so that they nearly assume its temperature. It was technically said of the *Alburkha,* the first of these vessels that ever went to sea, that she did not make "a cup of water," and we know that, in the course of her voyage up the Niger, she was the favorite vessel on this account, as well as from the circumstance of her being the healthier of the two vessels. The *Quorra,* that

accompanied her, very shortly lost two-thirds of her crew, while in the *Alburkha*, the sickness was nothing in comparison.

But iron hulls proved to be more than just healthy. In Britain, where timber was in short supply and costly, iron began to look like a viable economic alternative for vessel construction. The United States and Britain's North American colonies, unimpeded by any shortage of good shipbuilding timber, continued to construct wooden brigs, barks, and fast little schooners in vast numbers to compete commercially with Britain in the expanding international sea trade of the period.

In 1836 *Lloyd's Register* listed its first iron vessel, the ketch-rigged *Goliath*, followed two years later by the world's first full-rigged sailing vessel, appropriately named *Ironsides*. During the 1840s British shipbuilders were also discovering that riveted iron was considerably stronger than wood for hull construction, especially for very large vessels. Not only was iron stronger and less expensive than wood, but iron framing also took up less space than wood, resulting in more usable cargo space within the hull.

It came as no surprise then that when Isambard Brunel's revolutionary new 3,270-ton, 322-foot, six-masted ship SS *Great Britain* left her dry dock in 1843, she boasted a hull and frames constructed entirely of iron. Soon after her launch *Great Britain* became the first vessel with an iron hull to cross the Atlantic, beginning a career that would see her become a major conveyor of British emigrants to both America and Australia during her working life.

The success of *Great Britain* in 1843 essentially marked the true beginning of the age of iron ships, with total world tonnage reaching a peak about 1890 when iron's use began to decline and steel came into common use for hull construction.

Those who doubt the durability of iron for hull construction might consider visiting the port of Bristol, England, where they can view SS *Great Britain* sitting snugly in the same dry dock from which she was launched more than a century and a half before.

The Frank N. Thayer *Mutiny*

Midnight on January 2, 1886, found the Boston-registered *Frank N. Thayer* plowing Atlantic waters near latitude twenty-five degrees south, bound from Manila to New York with a cargo of 10,700 bales of hemp and twenty-four souls. On board were Captain Robert K. Clarke, his wife and nine-year-old daughter, and a multinational crew of nineteen, plus two Malayan seamen who had recently signed on at Manila for the return voyage to America.

Captain Clarke was no doubt pleased with the favorable winds driving his 1,592-ton, full-rigged vessel since rounding the Cape. But events were about to unfold aboard *Thayer* that would eventually see the total loss of the ship and her cargo and the deaths of seven of her crew.

Shortly after the midnight watch change, and without warning, the two Malay seamen drew their knives and began a bloody killing spree. They first attacked and stabbed the ship's carpenter, throwing his still-writhing body overboard. Immediately afterward they rushed and killed the stunned first and second mates, Mr. Holmer and Mr. Davies, who had been talking on deck. In rapid succession the mutineers went on to overpower and kill Maloney, the helmsman, and a lookout. The Malays viciously attacked the captain when he came on deck to investigate the commotion, inflicting on him a severe scalp wound and a near-fatal gash to his side from which his lung partially protruded. Bleeding and left for dead, Clarke managed to crawl back to his cabin and close and lock the door behind him before collapsing in front of his terrified wife and daughter.

Later, when Captain Clarke had recovered somewhat following the dressing of his wounds by his wife—who had managed to push the protruding lung back inside his chest wall—he opened the ship's arms locker and loaded two revolvers. As one of the mutineers looked down through the cabin's skylight at what was happening, Clarke fatally shot the man, who staggered over the side of the ship.

The remaining Malay, witnessing his fellow mutineer's demise, ran below to set fire to the cargo of baled hemp. The remaining members of the cowardly crew had, incredibly, barricaded themselves in the forecastle for safety and remained there until they saw smoke rising from the hold. The implicit danger of a fire at sea eventually prompted them to action. The crewmen left the forecastle and rushed down into the hold, where four of them were immediately attacked and wounded by the lone knife-wielding arsonist before he was struck and beaten back by a crewman wielding a fire ax. The Malay, mortally wounded by the ax blow, managed to elude his pursuers and escape through the after hatch. But rapidly bleeding to death and with nowhere to go, he let out a defiant yell before throwing himself over the side into the sea.

The captain soon recovered enough to direct the firefighting efforts. As a precaution, he ordered that his sextant, compass, and ship's chronometer be stowed aboard one of the ship's boats. When the heat and flames became intolerable and all hope of extinguishing the fire faded, the captain, his wife and child, and remaining crew abandoned the doomed *Thayer*. After a six-day ordeal in the open boat and using a makeshift sail of blankets, they finally made landfall at St. Helena, where the US consul took charge of the exhausted survivors.

The captain admitted to the consul and British newspaper reporters (who were always eager to report on a sensational mutiny) that he had punished the two new crewmen in late December, after *Thayer* had entered the South Atlantic, because they had proven to be "troublesome." It may have been this undisclosed punishment that provoked the Malays to bloody violence during the early hours of January 2.

However, had the journalists bothered to make telegraphic enquiries in the United States regarding Captain Clarke's history, they might have filed somewhat different stories. Captain Clarke had been convicted some thirteen years earlier of brutality toward his crew while he was master of the brig *Sunrise*, on a voyage from Liverpool to San Francisco—those actions having earned for him a hefty thousand-dollar fine and a year cooling his heels in the San Francisco jail.

39

Magnetic Compass Attracts Navigators

Technological development of the magnetic navigational compass has been ongoing for a very long time—perhaps as long as five millennia. Every navigational compass in use today is the product of continuous rich and varied refinements. Most compasses retain clues of their history, such as the stylized fleur-de-lis used to indicate north and the "points" still printed on the card.

The earliest rudimentary magnetic compass, like so many of humanity's more important technological breakthroughs, owes its development to the pressures and necessities of war. Chinese Emperor Huang-ti (2700 BCE) was pestered by a particularly persistent rebel leader whose forces had made a regular habit of harassing the emperor's troops in hit-and-run attacks, followed by successfully retreating to the safety of misty

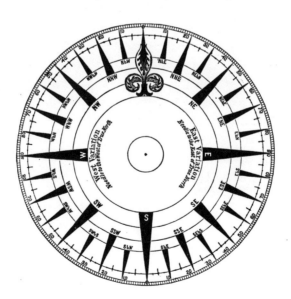

A compass rose, circa 1880. Note the fleur-de-lis emblem denoting north, a remnant of early French usage. Courtesy J. Gregory Dill (from his collection)

lowlands where they could effectively hide. What the emperor needed was a systematic, coordinated method of invading the rebel sanctuary, regardless of the area's persistent poor visibility.

The emperor's answer was found in a curious magnetic stone whose peculiar property, when it was suspended from a string, was that it would always point in the same direction once it had come to rest. Huang-ti ordered numerous of these rudimentary magnetic compasses to be mounted in wooden frames and made easily portable by mounting on wagons. Each wagon, followed by columns of imperial troops, moved forward on a broad coordinated front into the fog-shrouded enemy stronghold where they accurately and efficiently routed the enemy forces. Helpless against the systematic approach of the emperor's army, the rebel leader's army blindly stumbled about in zero visibility, unable to regroup or offer any kind of organized resistance, with the result that the rebel forces were eventually crushed.

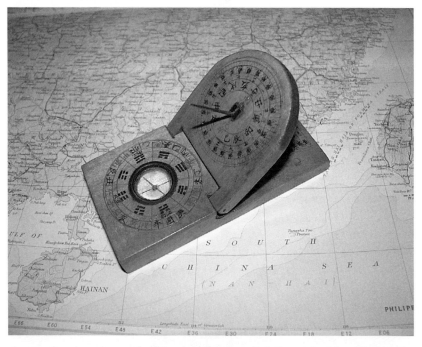

A copy of an ingenious early Chinese compass-sundial, the original possibly from the Ming dynasty (1368–1644). ©2005 by J. Gregory Dill

Lodestone (now called magnetite) was the bluish black to reddish mineral that solved the military problems of Huang-ti. The stone became highly prized for its predilection, when placed on a piece of wood floating on the surface of a bowl of water, for always presenting the same side of its mass toward the Pole Star. A good-quality stone offered an additional attraction for any lucky finder—he or she could expect to receive, in return for discovering it, the stone's equivalent weight in silver.

An anonymous later Chinese investigator found that he could magnetize a piece of iron wire (or needle) by touching it to a lodestone. The wire would then assume the stone's magnetic properties (albeit briefly). The magnetized wire could then be slipped into a piece of straw or stuck through a piece of cork and made to float upon a water surface to reveal north. Touching the needle to the lodestone was frequently required to maintain its north-seeking properties; the procedure became known as "feeding the needle."

Sailors in Europe may have been using crude magnetic compasses of Arab origin as early as 1000 CE. A thirteenth-century translation of a French account of the use of a marine compass by sailors records:

> . . . when in cloudy weather they can no longer profit by the light of the sun, or when the world is wrapped up in darkness of the shades of night and they are ignorant to what point of the compass their ship's course is directed, they touch the magnet with a needle, which is whirled round in a circle until, when its motion ceases, its point looks direct to north.

Floating a magnetized needle on a liquid surface was, however, not an easy thing to achieve, especially in a rolling sea. A pivot pin was eventually developed on which the needle could be mounted to rotate freely. This technological innovation was quickly followed in the West by the introduction of a compass card—a piece of round parchment about the size of a man's hand, mounted on the needle. The card's surface was marked with the points associated with the primary wind directions—north, east, south, and west, the cardinal points of the compass. These primary wind directions were further subdivided into halved winds, northeast, southeast, southwest, and northwest. Over time the compass card, or "compass rose" of the West, came to have thirty-two points. North was traditionally indicated on the card by a fleur-de-lis, likely because of the early use of marine compasses by the seamen from the ancient Aquitaine region of France. About the time of the Crusades, a cross symbol became the standard identifier for east, to indicate the direction of the Holy Land.

Between the thirteenth and fifteenth centuries marine compass design continued to steadily improve. By the beginning of the sixteenth century, Spanish navigator Martin Cortés had described in his book, *The Art of Navigation*, the construction of a contemporary marine compass that is surprisingly sophisticated by modern standards. It was a dry card type, utilizing a support cap and pivot constructed of a brass-like alloy set in gimbals, which were also built of the same alloy—the whole housed in a weatherproof wooden box with a hinged and sealed glass top.

The marine compass described by Cortés, and used by Spanish navigators in the monumental work of charting the waters of the New World, eventually became the principal design upon which all future marine magnetic compass innovations would be based.

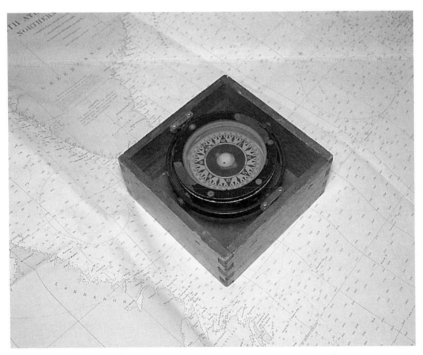

A small boat compass from the author's collection. ©2005 by J. Gregory Dill

10

Captain Voss and His Dugout Canoe

On July 6, 1901, one of the strangest sailing vessels ever to attempt a cruise around the world slipped away from the coast of Vancouver Island and out into the Pacific.

Christened *Tilikum* (a Nootka word meaning "friend"), the improbable little vessel carried aboard her an experienced master of merchant sailing ships, Captain John Claus Voss, and an imaginative Vancouver journalist-promoter, Norman Kenny Luxton.

Voss and Luxton met at Victoria in British Columbia and immediately became friends. As an experienced newspaperman, Luxton had been greatly impressed with the publicity generated by the recent successful voyage made around the world by Joshua Slocum. Luxton suggested that he and Voss should pool their respective professional talents to undertake a Slocum-like circumnavigation that would assure them a place in nautical history, and some serious money for their trouble. The cash would come from lectures and exhibitions at ports of call along the way and by publishing a book based on their adventures after the voyage. Voss readily agreed and set about searching for a suitable sailing craft for the venture.

Although their circumnavigation idea was hardly unique, Captain Voss's final selection of a vessel certainly was. He chose a thirty-eight-foot, West Coast aboriginal canoe—a "dugout" created by Native artisans almost a hundred years before from the trunk of a single red cedar. Voss and Luxton extensively modified their craft for ocean voyaging, raising her sides, installing a deck, and adding internal structural support. Included also were a keel, a rudder with cable steering, a cabin, and a cockpit. Three short masts were installed in *Tilikum*, and these were schooner-rigged. Water tanks were tucked under the cockpit, and a miniature wood-fired cookstove was shoehorned into the cabin on the starboard side.

On July 6 *Tilikum* and her crew of two began the great adventure, setting out from Vancouver Island. At sea Voss called upon his sailing expertise when experimenting with different sail combinations and relocating ballast, so that by the time *Tilikum* reached her first port of call, Penrhyn Island, Voss knew the handling capabilities of his boat very well. At Penrhyn friendly islanders welcomed and feted Voss and Luxton in grand style, providing them with entertainment and provisions.

Similar greetings met *Tilikum* at most islands on the voyage to Samoa. Differences, however, began to arise between Voss and Luxton— at one point, according to Luxton, Voss threatened to toss him into the ocean. By the time they reached Suva the enmity between the men had caused irreparable damage to their sailing partnership. That, and Luxton's unfortunate slowly deteriorating physical condition, meant a decision had to be made. Luxton finally left *Tilikum*, and the Voss–Luxton sailing partnership dissolved.

Before leaving Suva, Voss signed on a new mate, a competent Tasmanian seaman named Louis Bergent. But Bergent eventually fared worse than Luxton. When *Tilikum* arrived at Sydney, Australia, Voss was alone in the craft. He reported that Bergent had been washed overboard during the voyage, along with *Tilikum*'s only compass. After refitting *Tilikum*, Voss visited and lectured at several Australian ports. Disaster struck, however, at Melbourne when *Tilikum* was dropped and shattered while being lifted to a railcar for an inland tour. Undeterred, Voss patched up the splintered hull, then rigorously checked her seaworthiness before again continuing *Tilikum*'s tour.

Tilikum left Hobart, Tasmania, for a tour of New Zealand before finally sailing for the Coral Sea on August 17, 1902. Voss toured in South African waters for an extended period, then sailed for St. Helena and Pernambuco. After a refit in Brazil, *Tilikum* touched at the Azores, then headed for England, arriving three and a quarter years after leaving Victoria, British Columbia. More lecturing and exhibiting of *Tilikum* (always for a fee) followed. But Voss apparently tired of his rugged little sailing canoe, deciding not to continue with his lone circumnavigation, and he disposed of *Tilikum* before leaving England. Voss died in poverty in California, but not before publishing a book that included his sailing experiences aboard *Tilikum*.

By mere chance, a British Columbia naval man traveling in Britain in 1928 recognized *Tilikum*, abandoned and deteriorating on the Thames River mudflats. She was shipped home to Victoria and eventually restored. In 1965 *Tilikum* was adopted by the Maritime Museum of British Columbia, where she resides today, oddly appealing in her white paint and fresh canvas—a star artifact of the museum's collection that seems to lend credence to the words of poet William Blake when he wrote:

A fool sees not the same tree that the wise man sees.

Young Teazer *Gains Supernatural Status*

Duri ng the first months of the War of 1812 the privateer schooner *Teazer*, belonging to John Adams of New York, was seized by HMS *San Domingo*. Small schooners such as the armed *Teazer* were quickly being licensed by both America and Britain under letters of marque (see chapter 1), bestowing on masters of such private vessels the right to capture enemy merchant ships for profit.

In short order Adams replaced the lost *Teazer* with a new armed schooner that he christened *Young Teazer*. Maine-crafted from oak and Norway pine, *Young Teazer* displaced 124 tons, boasted a copper-clad hull, and carried five deck guns. She was a fast sailer, but in a flat calm could be rowed with sixteen oars at a speed of just over four knots. On her bow she carried a carved alligator figurehead—a showy display of her predatory intentions.

Frederick Johnson, *Young Teazer*'s first lieutenant, had also served in the former *Teazer*, where he had proven to be an unpopular officer with a particularly sour disposition. Johnson had been captured with *Teazer*'s crew and taken to Halifax as a prisoner of war. Enemy officers such as Johnson were considered "gentlemen" by the British and so were allowed parole—given the freedom of the town and a small money allowance for boardinghouse accommodation once they had signed a parole document in which they promised not to leave the confines of the town or take up arms against Britain again. Breaking the oath meant execution by hanging. Paroling of officers was certainly a much better deal than what befell the ordinary seamen from captured American, Spanish, or French vessels. These poor sailors were incarcerated in one of the Royal Navy's prison hulks in Halifax Harbor or at dismal and unhealthy Melville Island Military Prison, waiting sometimes years for freedom in a prisoner exchange. Johnson signed the parole document, but shortly thereafter was repatriated in a prisoner exchange.

On June 3, 1813, citizens of Portland turned out to watch *Young Teazer* hoist sail and shape a course for the dangerous coastal waters off Nova Scotia—dangerous because Britain had stationed at Halifax 106 naval vessels, including twenty massive seventy-four-gun ships of the line, as well as frigates and sloops-of-war. But for those crewing Adams's new privateer schooner, the financial incentive was well worth the risk. British prizes could, after disposition by sheriff's sale, net even an ordinary seaman the equivalent of ten years' wages for a few successful weeks of hot and hazardous cruising.

By June 11 Halifax newspapers were carrying stories of *Young Teazer*'s daring and profitable cruise, much to the embarrassment of senior Royal Navy staff. Orders were issued to capture this upstart American or destroy her on the water. Every British vessel ready for sea was sent out to patrol the coast, but whenever she was sighted *Young Teazer* always seemed to escape into a convenient fog bank. At one point the very fast Liverpool privateer *Sir John Sherbrooke* gave chase, but lost the faster American in the persistent south shore mists. *Young Teazer* continued capturing and sending rich prizes back to New England and New York, but the little armed privateer's luck was about to change.

By midafternoon of June 20, 1813, the frigate HMS *La Hogue* had spotted *Young Teazer* and managed to bottle her up in Mahone Bay. There was no fog that day to hide in as the late-afternoon wind began to fail. The American set out her oars in the dying breeze, but had nowhere to go. *La Hogue*—dead in the water, but with *Young Teazer* in sight—anchored and immediately sent off five heavily armed ship's boats toward the privateer. On board *Young Teazer* the captain considered his only two options: He could choose to fight it out or abandon his schooner and row his ship's boat to shore in an attempt to escape capture. While the captain pondered his decision, Lieutenant Johnson took matters into his own hands, making a panicked and particularly selfish decision to end the dilemma. Knowing that he would swing from the nearest yardarm for breaking his parole if taken prisoner again, Johnson rushed down into the galley, took a ladle of glowing coals from the stove, and headed to the schooner's powder magazine.

The resulting explosion rattled windows more than ten miles away. Twenty-eight of the thirty-six crew, including Johnson, were killed outright in the blast. Surprisingly, part of the sturdy hull of *Teazer* remained afloat after the rest of her had burned to the waterline. Farmers and townspeople who had gathered on the shore to watch the fight were shaken by what they had witnessed. The bystanders, along with fishermen who were on the bay at the time, collected the badly burned survivors, taking them into their homes for care. Others gathered up what grisly human remains they could find; the following day a local Lutheran clergyman conducted a burial service for the dead, in German. Part of *Young Teazer*'s oak keelson was salvaged and from it was constructed a cross that is still displayed at a local church.

Johnson's fateful decision to destroy his own vessel later caused consternation and angry debate back in America. One indignant New York newspaper editor suggested of Lieutenant Johnson that ". . . he must have been possessed of the disposition of a devil to plunge such a number of his friends into eternity, who had parents, wives and children to mourn their untimely fate . . ."

But that was not the end of the tale of *Young Teazer* and her destruction at the hands of her own first officer. Exactly one year to the date of *Young Teazer*'s demise, fishermen working out on Mahone Bay spied what appeared to be a flaming wreck of a schooner drifting down upon them, out of a fog bank. As they watched in horror, fearing the blazing craft would set their own boats afire, the burning schooner disappeared in a brilliant flash of light. That event spawned a maritime tradition— that of a ghostly apparition of a bold Yankee schooner with raked masts that still regularly slips out of the fogs of Mahone Bay to drift a few minutes among yachts and fishing craft, before disappearing in a silent, fiery flash that has become known as the Teazer Light.

Bad Poetry, Barometers, and Reckoning the Weather

When it is evening, ye say, it will be fair weather; for the sky is red.

And in the morning, it will be foul weather to day; for the sky is red and lowering.

—MATTHEW 16:2–3

To the sailor, the above bit of biblical weather advice is better known in the following rhyme:

A red sky in the morning, sailors take warning;
A red sky at night is a sailor's delight.

For millennia intelligent sailors tried to forecast the weather via the appearance of the sky and cloud formations, in conjunction with the fluctuations in wind speed and direction. This knowledge was codified in simple rhymes and passed along to generations of apprentice seamen.

By the beginning of the nineteenth century new sailors were still learning many weather rhymes to help them make correct choices at sea—everything from what sail combinations their vessel should be carrying for expected weather conditions to when a pump watch should be set, as evidenced by the following rhymes:

When rain comes before the wind,
halyard, sheets, and braces mind.

When wind comes before the rain,
soon you may make sail again.
and,

When the porpoise jumps,
Stand by your pumps.

But a technical revolution was taking place in weather prediction between the beginning and end of the nineteenth century, and this revolution began to show up in "modernized" weather rhymes:

At sea with low and falling glass,
soundly sleeps the careless ass.
Only when it's high and rising,
truly rests a careful wise one.

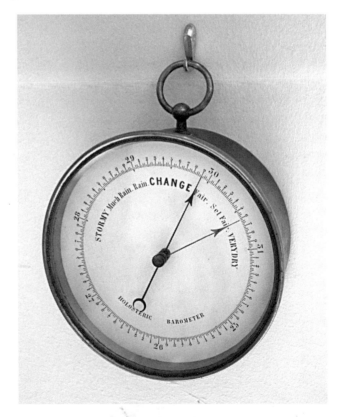

This brass barometer from the author's collection, a French design of 1888, still works flawlessly despite never having been opened for servicing.
©2003 by
J. Gregory Dill

The "glass" referred to above was of course the glass-tubed mercury barometer, a tool that, when combined with his well-worn weather wit, might forewarn a seaman of future foul weather. But it was the development of the radical new aneroid barometer in 1844 that gave seamen a more valuable weather instrument. The word *aneroid*, derived from Greek words meaning "not of fluid form," was touted by one Captain Lecky in his massive, 777-page book *Wrinkles in Practical Navigation* (1881). He noted that the aneroid barometer "is by far the better instrument for use afloat. It is more portable, and occupies much less room . . . and is more sensitive than the mercurial barometer, and at all times—more especially in heavy weather—easier to read."

Since it was more accurate and much easier to read, it became possible for very minute changes in pressure to be more readily detected by the observant captain reading his aneroid barometer's finely divided analog scale. He began to notice that small changes in pressure seemed always to occur when his ship tacked and soon learned that in the Northern Hemisphere (in all wind conditions except near the equator), tacking to starboard would take his ship toward a higher barometer, while tacking to port would take it toward a lower one.

By the end of the nineteenth century some of the complicated weather mechanisms driving storm (and specifically hurricane) formation and track were beginning to be better understood, thanks to the aneroid barometer. The US Navy's Hydrographic Office *Publication 86* (1901) offered the following nonrhyming recommendations to masters using aneroid barometers (based on decades of logged information) for preparing a vessel ahead of an approaching hurricane:

> A vessel suspecting the dangerous proximity of a hurricane should lie-to for a time on the starboard tack to locate the center by observing shifts of the wind and the behavior of the barometer. If the former holds steady and increases in force, while the latter falls rapidly, say at a rate greater than 0.03 of an inch per hour, the vessel is probably on the track of the storm.

But even with such a valuable and growing body of scientific weather knowledge available at the close of the nineteenth century, some seamen still chose to fall back on the security of those bad poetic musings for guidance in certain waters. One humorous, if pessimistic, example is an Irish variation on that old jingle for remembering the number of days in each month; this version relates to the weather a seaman can expect to encounter near the coasts of Ireland—barometer be damned:

Dirty days hath September,
April, June and November.
From January up to May,
the rain it cometh every day.
All the rest have thirty-one
without a blessed gleam of sun;
and if any of them had two and thirty,
they'd be just as wet and twice as dirty.

Figurehead Function and Fashion

Visit any large maritime museum, and somewhere among the exhibits and displays you can expect to find at least one intricately carved and painted figurehead from some long-vanished sailing vessel.

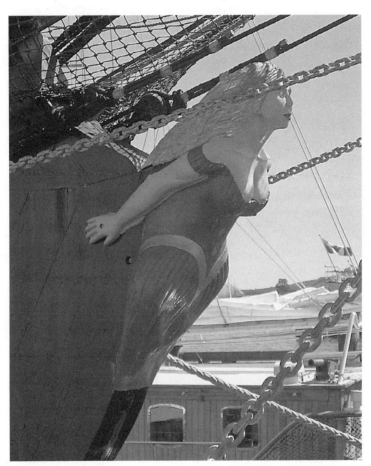

A mermaid figurehead on the bow of a present-day sailing vessel.
©2005 by J. Gregory Dill

A figurehead, in the marine sense, is defined by the *Oxford International Dictionary* (1958) as "A piece of carving, usually a bust or figure, placed over the cutwater of a ship." The reasons for attaching this embellishment to the bow are lost in prehistory, but in his book *Ships' Figureheads*, Peter Norton mentions rock carvings found in caves on Lake Onega in Russia showing what appears to be the real heads of animals mounted on the bows of early boats of that area.

Figurehead use may have originated as a religious or mythological symbol employed to protect a ship from storms or voracious sea creatures. It may also have been an attempt to give eyes to a vessel to allow it to "see" its way during a voyage—making a figurehead, in a sense, a kind of supernatural navigational instrument. An early recorded reference of possible figurehead use can be found in Acts 28:11 of the Bible when Paul the Apostle notes, ". . . after three months we departed in a ship of Alexandria [Egypt], which had wintered on the isle [Malta], whose sign was Castor and Pollux." Castor and Pollux were mythological twin sons of Zeus and were supposed to protect seamen from harm. The "sign" that Paul saw was almost certainly a carved or painted image of the twin gods mounted at the bow of the ship.

Through the centuries sea-roving Egyptians, Phoenicians, Greeks, Romans, and Vikings used numerous carved animal images as figureheads. An early merchant vessel might have carried on her stempost the carved head of a swan or crane, in the hope that the gracefulness or swiftness characteristic of the chosen bird might be imparted to the ship. Diving birds such as cormorants and kingfishers seem not to have been popular, for obvious reasons. A vessel of war would have carried something a bit more aggressive—say, the head of a wild boar, bull, or serpent—to intimidate crews of enemy vessels. Horses seem to have been a particular favorite of Phoenician shipowners.

When William the Conqueror sailed from Normandy in 1066 to subjugate England, his ship carried a sculpted lion's head, a departure from the usual dragon or serpent's image popular in Northern Europe at the time. The lion figurehead remained a favorite, gracing numerous English fighting ships during the next eight hundred years. As time passed, European advancements in ship design and building techniques changed how figureheads were mounted. Development of the carrack design, for instance, meant the forward part of the forecastle could be more easily incorporated into a favorite creature's head or body.

Sir Francis Drake, Queen Elizabeth I's "royal pirate," had a carved, golden effigy of a fleet-footed red deer mounted on his ship, *Golden*

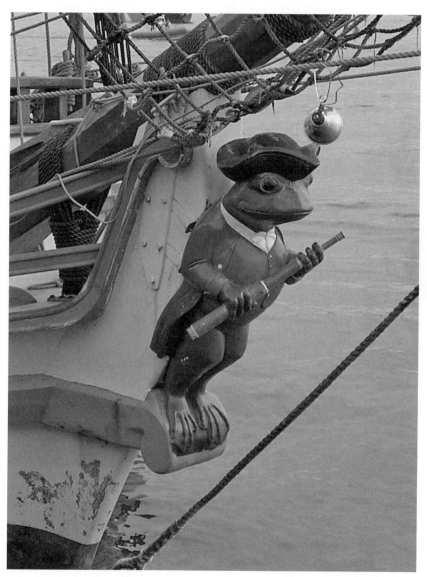

A frog figurehead on the bow of a ship. ©2005 by J. Gregory Dill

Hind—a symbol he probably hoped would engender his vessel with a swiftness his Spanish prey could not possibly hope to outrun. The Spanish, on the other hand, encumbered by sluggish, lumbering treasure ships, felt the sensible course to follow to avoid El Draco's piratical molestations was to seek Divine Intervention—employing figureheads depicting saints and the Holy Trinity for protection.

In America figurehead art initially imitated those styles and themes popular in England. For instance, during the American Revolution the US Frigate *Raleigh* sported a finely rendered figurehead of Sir Walter himself, in war-like pose, an irony probably not lost on the British enemy. The young republic soon began producing its own unique style of ship art, incorporating American themes such as Indian warriors, presidents, and native animals. Some shipowners chose to immortalize their wives, daughters, and sisters by having them sit for marine artists who produced sometimes beautiful (and just as often mundane) figureheads to decorate a family-owned vessel named for the lucky female.

A carving typical of a mid-nineteenth-century female subject graces the replica bark *Jeanie Johnson*, which recently completed a commemorative voyage from Ireland to North America celebrating her namesake's cruises during which thousands of Irish emigrants were brought to the New World. Many mariners actually credited the charm of buxom female figureheads like that of *Jeanie Johnson* with the capacity to calm the most turbulent waters.

Sadly, the advent of iron and steam-powered ships heralded a steady decline in the production of marine figurehead art. Today we are fortunate to be able view a vintage figurehead in a museum display or to glimpse a rare but authentic "working" figurehead—one displayed on the prow of a restored sailing ship, or mounted sedately on the bow of a replica vessel such as *Jeanie Johnson*.

What Shall We Do with a Drunken Sailor?

Once, while decanting a bottle of Chianti, Italian sailor and revolutionary Giuseppe Garibaldi was heard to remark, "Bacchus has drowned more men than Neptune."

That, unfortunately, sums up how most of the world has always viewed the poor sailor—as a drunkard. Throughout recorded history the public has held the character of the sailor in a less-than-charitable light, because most landlubbers have only ever seen him at his worst— while ashore. A vision of the sea-weary sailor, seriously inebriated, or working hard at becoming so, brawling in the harborside taverns, pubs, and bars of the world, or roaming the streets in groups, singing off-color songs and in constant search of demon drink and the fellowship of ladies of besmirched virtue, was as universal among the good citizens of fifteenth-century Genoa as it was to those living through the gold rush days of San Francisco. And the cry *the fleet's in* brought to mothers of every era shocking visions of soused seamen seeking out their blossoming daughters who, if time allowed, would be briskly bundled off to the care of maiden aunts, well inland. The biased and negative stereotype of the intemperate mariner can even be seen in the work of Hans Holbein, that celebrated sixteenth-century artist whose painting *Ship with Armed Men* clearly portrays sailors on a vessel under sail, drinking heavily in every corner of their ship and cavorting with a prostitute. Even the *American Coast Pilot* of 1817 contributed to the assault on the sailor's character by warning its readers en route to the port of Savannah, Georgia:

> . . . masters and commanders of vessels trading to this province are often greatly distressed by the neglect or desertion of their seamen, which is in general occasioned by such seamen being harboured and entertained by and running into debt with the keepers of taverns and tippling houses, and ill disposed persons, to the great detriment and hindrance of trade.

Perhaps now is the time for the modern follower of the sea to exude a more temperate and cultured demeanor, especially when frequenting dockside watering holes. Share a meaningful dialogue with your drinking companions and others on some important topic—the importance of moral rectitude in contemporary government, for instance. And above all, avoid spitting on the floor!

Together, with a little thought and tact, sailors just might be able to turn the tide of public opinion in favor of the sailing fraternity.

I'll drink to that!

15

Who Was Henry Morgan?

oogle the words "Captain Morgan," and among the search results you will find this famous name gracing a popular rum label, a retreat in Belize, a cruise line in Malta, and even a pub in the Polish port city of Gdansk.

Such is the universal appeal of the flamboyant character who, for most of the world, personifies the image of a freebooting, swashbuckling buccaneer—Sir Henry Morgan. But the real Morgan is decidedly more difficult to separate from the myth.

Morgan began life in Monmouthshire, Wales, in 1635, evidently born into a good family with old connections to the English court. He left his native Wales about 1655 to become a member of an English military expedition that later seized the strategic Caribbean island of Jamaica from Spain. In 1663 Morgan was part of an English force that successfully captured the colonial city of Santiago de Cuba, a major administrative and provisions base for protecting Spanish power in the Caribbean.

It might be more correct to describe Morgan as a licensed privateer of sorts, rather than a pirate, although he certainly associated with real pirates on a more or less regular basis. The governor of Jamaica, Sir Thomas Modyford, issued Morgan a letter of marque (see chapter 1) in 1670 as England's response to Spain's instructions to her West Indies governors to wage war on British possessions. This document reads in part:

> Whereas Don Pedro Bayona de Villa Nueva, Captain General of the Province of Paraguay and Governor of the City of St. Jago de Cuba and its Provinces, hath . . . lately in the most hostile and barbarous manner landed his men on the north side of the Island [of Jamaica], and entered a small way into the country, firing all the Houses they came at, killing or taking Prisoners all the inhabitants they could meet with . . .

The wordy document continues, showing the great faith Modyford had in Morgan's ability:

> In discharge of the great trust which His Gracious Majesty hath placed in me, I do by virtue of full Power and Authority of such cases from His Royal Highness, James Duke of York, His Majesties Lord High Admiral, derived unto me, and out of the great confidence I have in the good conduct, courage, and fidelity of you the said Henry Morgan to be Admiral and Commander in Chief of all Ships, Barques, and other Vessels now fitted out . . .

Morgan's orders were perfectly clear and quite legal—he was to harass the Spanish at every turn. In 1671 he sailed on his most audacious cruise with a flotilla of thirty-nine ships carrying two thousand men, including known pirates, to the coast of the Isthmus of Darien (the present-day Isthmus of Panama) in Central America. After landing, Morgan marched part of his force across the isthmus, where he successfully attacked and looted Panama in reprisal for the Spanish attacks on Jamaica. When Morgan returned to Port Royal to a hero's welcome, he carried with him a fortune in personally looted treasure. Unfortunately, delayed word of his exploits at Panama had reached London just as King Charles II chose to seek improved relations with Spain. The English king decided to denounce the Panama raid to appease the Spanish court, and Morgan was arrested, as was Governor Modyford who had issued Morgan his credentials.

Morgan was summoned to England, but remarkably was not tried or punished after his arrival. He remained at large to charm the society ladies of London and the royal court in general and easily gained the ear of the king. In fact, Morgan got on so well with his monarch that Charles not only forgave him all his past actions, but also knighted him. When relations with Spain again began to sour, Charles sent Sir Henry home to Jamaica as colonel and deputy governor of the island, convinced no doubt that Morgan was the best man with whom to entrust the profitable island's security.

Once back in Jamaica, Morgan settled easily into the comfortable life of chief gentleman at the island's capital, Port Royal. He did not, however, hesitate to foster the illegal practices of his former pirate friends, while outwardly appearing to suppress those same associates' illicit activities. This continued up until his death on August 25, 1688. Captain Lawrence Wright of the frigate HMS *Assistance* recorded the event in his diary:

> This day about eleven hours noon Sir Henry Morgan died, and the 26th was brought over from Passage-fort to the King's house at Port Royal, from thence to the Church, and after a sermon was carried to the Pallisadoes and there buried. All the forts fired an equal number of guns; we fired two and twenty, and after we and the Drake had fired, all the merchant-men fired.

Sir Henry Morgan died a much-respected citizen and hero, unaware that his name would remain a household word more than three centuries after his death—a name that would lend itself to advertising everything from liquor to tourist travel, and be the catalyst for countless myths and tales of buried booty and bold, bloody buccaneers.

Minor Collision Destroys Port

For more than 250 years the histories of the port cities of Boston and Halifax have been irrevocably linked and intertwined. But one shared bit of history that may not be as well known as it should links the annual lighting of a giant Christmas tree at Boston's Prudential Center with a marine collision that occurred nearly a century ago, in the Narrows of Halifax Harbor.

A crisp, clear morning greeted Halifax dockworkers as they made their way to work on December 6, 1917. Because World War I was still

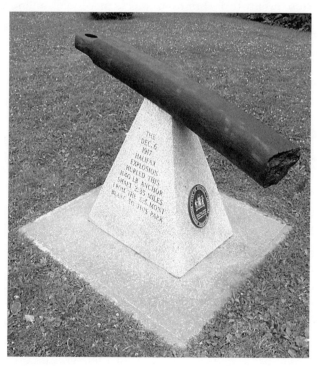

This 1,140-pound anchor shaft from one of Mont Blanc's *bow anchors was thrown more than two miles by the force of the explosion.* ©2003 by J. Gregory Dill

raging in Europe, the port found itself extremely busy handling ships, war matériel, and men, just as it had during all of the British Empire's wars since the fall of Quebec in 1759. Few Haligonians with a view of the harbor that morning would have taken much notice of the unmooring, shortly after 8 AM, of a neutral Norwegian ship, the former whaler SS *Imo* (Captain Hakkon From). *Imo* was heading to New York to pick up humanitarian supplies for civilian victims of the war in Europe. Large letters on *Imo*'s topsides proclaimed BELGIUM RELIEF, in the hope the message would keep prowling German submarines from sinking her.

Farther up the harbor another vessel, the rusty Marseilles-registered munitions ship *Mont Blanc* (Captain A. Le Medec) was proceeding in the opposite direction, having arrived earlier from New York. *Mont Blanc*'s cargo was the complete opposite of the beneficent freight *Imo* had recently carried, for stowed on board the French ship was a cargo capable of destroying human life—thirty-five tons of benzene, ten tons of gun cotton, twenty-three hundred tons of picric acid, ammunition for her own guns, and the unthinkable—nearly two hundred tons of trinitrotoluene, better known as TNT. *Mont Blanc* was, in fact, little more than a floating bomb.

As *Imo* steered into the natural constriction of the harbor called the Narrows, she kept a course tight to the Dartmouth side of the passage. The two ships on opposing tracks soon confronted each other, and in the first of a series of signals exchanged between the ships' bridges, *Imo*'s captain indicated his intention to keep his course more to port (shoreward). A further flurry of signals followed until the vessels were dangerously close to each other. The two captains decided to take evasive action simultaneously, virtually ensuring a collision. Le Medec turned *Mont Blanc* hard to port, intending to pass *Imo* starboard-to-starboard, rather than the customary port-to-port. At the same instant Captain From called for "full astern" on *Imo*'s engine telegraph, causing her bows to swing out across *Mont Blanc*'s track.

Neither ship sustained major damage in the ensuing low-speed impact, but sparks from the collision quickly ignited damaged and leaking drums stored on *Mont Blanc*'s deck. As the fire spread, the entire crew of *Mont Blanc* abandoned ship, rowing for their lives toward the Dartmouth shore. The blazing, crewless *Mont Blanc* drifted lazily across the Narrows toward the Halifax piers, passing near enough to one to set its tarred timbers ablaze. At 9:05 AM, as a city fire brigade attempted to bring the pier blaze under control, the fire aboard *Mont Blanc* reached the deadly store of TNT deep in the hold of the ship. The ensuing explosion would go down in history as the greatest human-made explosion until the atom bombing of Hiroshima.

The effect was immediate and devastating. Sixteen hundred citizens of Halifax were killed outright. The number of injured amounted to just under ten thousand, while the northern part of the city had been reduced to a smoldering, blackened wasteland. *Mont Blanc* had disintegrated into steel splinters that rained down for miles around. One of her anchor shanks weighing 1,140 pounds was thrown more than two miles to the opposite side of the peninsula on which the city stands—passing over the graveyard where many of the victims of another marine collision, the *Titanic*, had been buried five years earlier.

Word of the tragedy was relayed quickly up and down the Atlantic seaboard by railway telegraph. The first major humanitarian response to news of the disaster came from Halifax's old maritime nemesis—the port of Boston. By chance, the governor of Massachusetts was in a telegraph office when the news arrived. Only nine hours after the explosion, the state government and citizens of Boston had organized a massive relief operation, sending the first of a series of trains carrying food, building materials, medical supplies, and doctors north to battered Halifax. The trains also included special railcars outfitted with electrical generators and operating rooms to treat the thousands of wounded swamping Halifax hospitals.

Many in Halifax blamed German agents for the explosion, although no evidence of a plot has ever been uncovered. That rumor has subsided with the passage of time, but not forgotten is the timely and generous assistance provided by Boston and the commonwealth of Massachusetts. Each year since the devastating marine disaster, Halifax has sent a special Christmas "thank-you" to the citizens of Boston—a giant Nova Scotia fir tree to act as the centerpiece of Boston's annual Christmas celebrations.

17

Of Mermaids and Mariners

Just how long did a sailor have to be at sea before a passing manatee, seal, or dolphin began to take on the appearance of the girl next door? And was this vision of an alluring creature, half woman and half mackerel, simply a product of agitated hormones induced by months or years of being deprived of intimate female companionship? Could a dubious bit of ship's biscuit, a portion of salt pork well past its due date, or one too many tokes on a favorite piece of hemp hawser have been contributing factors also? Without doubt, some combination of the preceding must have conspired to create in the sailor's mind the miraculous transformation of an ordinary sea mammal into the sensual and desirable mermaid.

The *Oxford International Dictionary* says mermaids are "an imaginary species of beings, supposed to inhabit the sea, and to have the head and trunk of a woman, ending in a tail of a fish or cetacean." However one defines these beguiling creatures, they seem to have been teasing mariners for more than twenty centuries, with every seagoing culture having recorded their existence.

The Greeks wrote of "Nereids" who lived in the sea and would foretell a mariner's future—a definite plus for the sailor who had consulted one before an evening of rolling dice with his shipmates. A legend of a mermaid comes down to us from the sixth-century Christian colony on Iona, an isolated island off the Scottish west coast, founded by Saint Colomba (one of the first men reported to have seen the Loch Ness monster). It seems Saint Colomba had a problem with one of his monks who, while walking alone on the island's rocky shore, encountered a mermaid who wished to obtain a human soul. This lonely and amorous monk evidently fell head-over-sandals for his scaly friend, requiring the monastery's CEO to institute damage-control measures to protect the colony's good name.

Mermaid stories have also appeared in the early history of the New World. Christopher Columbus recorded seeing mermaids playing about his vessel off the coast of Guyana, South America, in 1493. But the Admiral of the Ocean Sea seems to have been little impressed with their beauty, recording in his log that they "were not so faire as they are painted." Back in Europe, a Dane named Busseus wrote of a merman having been captured by two Norwegian noblemen in a fishing net in Bergen Fjord. As the creature was hauled aboard, it cursed its captors and threatened (apparently in flawless Norwegian) to send their tiny boat to the bottom of the fjord if they did not immediately release him. Not wishing to chance the loss of their vessel, or having to carry such a wild story back to their marine insurance agents, the highborn piscators gingerly slipped their cursing catch back into the depths.

Endless legends of mermaids have been generated by the minds of those isolated in some way from the mainstream culture, whether away at sea or living on secluded islands. The myths seem likely to continue, destined to live on in the minds of future celestial navigators engaged in lonely voyages to distant parts of our star system, who might be expected to conjure up mermaid- or merman-like companions to help ease the isolation and boredom of the trip—curious little creatures, perhaps half human and half rocket thruster.

18

The Gulf Stream (Part One)

The Gulf Stream, or more correctly the North Equatorial Current, has its origins in the Caribbean Sea. There, seawater absorbs the heat of the sun and expands to flow into the Gulf of Mexico, where it undergoes additional heating and further expansion until it finally escapes through the Straits of Florida, between Florida and Cuba, as a "river in the ocean." This river of warm water varies in width from forty to fifty miles as it flows northeast along the Atlantic coast of the United States to as far north as the Grand Banks of Newfoundland, before continuing on across the Atlantic to Northern Europe, bringing with it a relatively temperate climate to those lands.

The presence of the stream had been noted from at least the time of the Spanish explorer Juan Ponce de León in the fifteenth century. Then, in the eighteenth century, Herr Doktor Fahrenheit suggested that his scientific invention for measuring temperature, the Fahrenheit thermometer, might be of assistance to ships' captains in navigating at sea, especially through the "river in the sea."

Statesman, entrepreneur, and scientist Benjamin Franklin took the good doctor's advice and decided to conduct his own investigations into the mysterious "river" that Franklin named the Gulf Stream. Franklin was engaged in a number of diplomatic missions across the Atlantic just prior to the American Revolution in an attempt to wring political concessions from America's British masters. Later he sailed to France to court French sentiment and support for America's push for independence. Franklin was no sailor, and he suffered long and frequently from bouts of seasickness on those voyages. But despite his uncomfortable ocean crossings, Franklin could not resist satisfying his scientific curiosity when his ship approached the Gulf Stream. During those times he left his diplomatic paperwork in his cabin and, though weak from the effects of the ship's motion, struggled to the weather deck to conduct temperature measurements. He trailed a thermometer (tied to the end of a piece of string) from the side of the ship, made copious observations of temperature variations, then recorded them carefully in detailed notes that would later be used to help map a portion of the course of the Gulf Stream.

In June 1791 Captain William Billings of Philadelphia followed Franklin's lead and took temperature readings near thirty-nine degrees north and fifty-six degrees west. He reported a drop in water temperature of almost ten degrees as his ship progressed abreast of Newfoundland's Grand Banks. Franklin had made similar observations at almost the same spot in 1776, as did Jonathan Williams in November 1789. Pondering these recorded tidbits of information led Williams to conclude that a navigator could discover his approach toward dangerous shoals or his entrance into the Gulf Stream "by attentively examining the temperature of the sea; the water over banks and shoals being colder than that of the deep ocean."

Williams used his own and Franklin's data in a book titled *Thermometrical Navigation* published in 1799, in which he urged navigators, when approaching the North American coast, to have available two matched thermometers—one attached to a shaded area on deck to measure the air temperature, and the other trailed behind the vessel to measure water temperature. By recording and comparing the air and water temperatures every two hours, the navigator could, according to Williams, determine when his ship entered and exited the Gulf Stream. This knowledge would also permit the navigator to make allowance for the distance his vessel would be set northward by multiplying the time while in the stream by the velocity of the current. Williams suggested this procedure could shorten voyage time from Britain to America by as much as five days and would be particularly useful if the navigator had been unable to take a sextant altitude of the sun for several days.

Williams's navigational thermometer method suggests a novel addition that organizers of the famous annual Marion-Bermuda Cruising Yacht Race might wish to consider incorporating in their race rules—offering a "time bonus" to those entrants who decide to sail to Bermuda, navigating by thermometer alone.

The Gulf Stream (Part Two)

As mentioned in The Gulf Stream (Part One), the first investigator to really seriously study the nature of the Gulf Stream was Benjamin Franklin. It seemed fitting, then, that when a high-tech undersea vessel, first designated *PX-15*, was purposely built to intimately study that curious "river in the ocean" almost two centuries after the death of that celebrated American statesman, philosopher, and scientist, the name chosen for the craft would be *Ben Franklin.*

Ben Franklin was laid down in Switzerland in 1966 and completed two years later, with funding from Grumman Corporation and the National Aeronautics and Space Administration. What possible interest could Grumman and NASA have in a vehicle that could navigate the depths of the oceans? Obviously, lessons learned in designing environments to support human life in a hostile, isolated environment could be applied successfully to future spacecraft design.

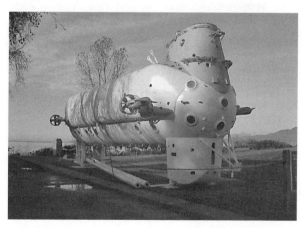

The 130-ton PX-15, *better known as* Ben Franklin, *sits high and dry near the Vancouver Maritime Museum. The four side-mounted electric motors, twenty-five horsepower each, were used only for maneuvering during the Gulf Stream Drift Mission.* ©2003 by J. Gregory Dill

Like her namesake, *Franklin* was of a slightly rotund appearance, but solid. She had a displacement of 132 tons, measured almost fifty feet from stem to stern, had a twenty-two-foot beam, and could accommodate modestly well a captain and crew of five, none of whom should suffer seriously from claustrophobia. The vessel's structure and unique design benefited from the considerable experience of the famous Piccard family of France, the original idea for the craft having taken root in the fertile and adventurous mind of French explorer Jacques Piccard.

Piccard had earlier, with his father, designed and built a small submersible craft for ocean exploration, and later made a world record dive to the deepest area in the world's oceans, almost thirty-six thousand feet down in the Marianas Trench, in 1960 in the bathyscaphe *Trieste.*

Franklin was destined to fulfill a goal of studying the Gulf Stream from within, in a project known as the Gulf Stream Drift Mission—a planned passive voyage calling for the insertion of the vessel into the Gulf Stream, where she would drift, submerged, in the flow for thirty days. With the vessel's forward movement dependent upon the movement of the stream, *Franklin* was unlike any conventional submarine that depends on powered forward movement to maintain depth. Since she was meant to simply drift along, submerged, navigation would be confined to controlling depth and avoiding underwater obstructions such as coral heads and shipwrecks. Maneuvering was to be accomplished by using four articulated electric motors, twenty-five horsepower each, arranged along the sides of the vessel and supplied with power by batteries stowed in the keel. Emergency surfacing, if it became necessary, would be accomplished by dumping six tons of steel shot carried as ballast.

The adventure began on France's Independence Day, July 14, 1969, off Palm Beach in Florida. Jacques Piccard, Captain Don Kazimir (an experienced submariner), and four other intrepid international specialist crewmen, including a NASA observer along for the trip to monitor human responses within an isolated environment, boarded *Franklin.* There has been no confirmation of whether the ghost of scientist Benjamin Franklin went along for the cruise, but if his spirit were present in the damp submersible laboratory, it would probably have appreciated the smooth passage. The crew undertook an intensive study of the oceanographic mysteries of the Gulf Stream and recorded the psychological and physical effects on humans confined for a month in an isolated steel cylinder. Tabs were kept on *Franklin*'s position by an accompanying support ship on the surface and US Navy patrol aircraft. The project also gave the stream's marine life its first decent chance to observe humans up close. Attracted by light escaping from the vessel's viewing ports, sharks, swordfish, tuna, squid, and giant jellyfish inquisitively ogled the large white-and-yellow alien object and the curious parasitic life-forms infesting the interior of *Ben Franklin*.

When the highly successful drifting voyage finally terminated without incident thirty days later, *Franklin* and her crew had covered almost fifteen hundred miles at an average speed of just under fifty miles per day and had collected valuable data that would prove of particular interest to those researching in the areas of oceanography and space travel.

So why have you never heard of the Gulf Stream Drift Mission? Most likely because just two days after *Ben Franklin* slipped beneath the waters of the stream to begin her voyage of discovery, the world media's attention had become focused exclusively on another notable navigational project in which both Grumman and NASA also had a stake—that being the *Apollo 11* mission that ultimately succeeded in placing the first human on the surface of the moon.

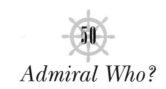

Admiral Who?

What a heavy burden is a name that has become too famous.

—VOLTAIRE

When Pavel Stepanovich Nakhimov was born in Gorodok in 1802, few of the inhabitants of that tiny Russian village 120 miles west of Moscow could have guessed that this native son's name would eventually be associated with bad-luck ships.

Pavel Nakhimov first entered Russian history books in 1853 when, as admiral of a squadron of Russia's Black Sea Fleet, he successfully blockaded most of the Turkish navy at Sinope, before he proceeded to totally destroy it. His name quickly became a household word across the czar's realm. Perhaps predictably, Nakhimov's popularity precipitated a proliferation of "baby Pavels" as parents proudly proclaimed their newborn male progeny named for the hero of Sinope.

When the combined forces of Britain, France, and Turkey attacked the port city of Sevastopol (in the Russian Crimea) in 1854–55, it was left to the freshly minted national celebrity (now commander of the port and military governor) to save the day. Nakhimov's strategy for defending the city and the Russian navy's main Black Sea base at Sevastopol proved brilliant. But on one of his many visits to inspect Russian defensive positions, he was unlucky enough to be struck by a British sniper's bullet and killed. The fallen hero's name now assumed a mythic quality in Russia, much as Admiral Horatio Nelson's had fifty years earlier in Britain. Nakhimov's name quickly lent itself to Russian monuments, schools, public buildings, medals of bravery, and, not surprisingly, Russian ships.

One of these, the cruiser *Admiral Nakhimov,* was launched in 1885 and served in the Russian Imperial Navy during the Russo-Japanese War of 1904–05. It was during this conflict that the cruiser suffered an ignominious end when, after being struck and disabled by a Japanese torpedo, her crew scuttled her to prevent the cruiser's capture by enemy forces.

Another luckless ship was destined to share the same watery fate as that Russian naval cruiser, some eighty years later. She began life as the German luxury liner SS *Berlin*, launched at Bremen in 1925. *Berlin* had a troubled later life. In 1939 a deadly explosion in the boiler room killed nine of *Berlin*'s crew. She was sent for repairs, but while in dry dock Adolf Hitler's Nazi government decided she would be converted to a hospital ship, in preparation for war duty. *Berlin* fared reasonably well until near the end of the conflict, when she was sunk after striking a mine. Given the history of this ship and her condition after the war, it was surprising that the Soviet government should have decided to claim the sunken hulk as a war prize. *Berlin* was raised, refurbished, and then returned to passenger configuration for Soviet use. Understandably, the Kremlin wanted to give the resurrected German passenger liner a new name. *Berlin* became *Admiral Nakhimov*.

So the former *Berlin*, raised from a watery grave after having suffered two deadly explosions, was given the name of another vessel that had sunk. Evidently superstition was not part of the Soviet psyche in the years following World War II. In fact, *Admiral Nakhimov*, alias *Berlin*, went about her duties as a Soviet cruise ship without serious incident until the night of August 31, 1986. As Captain V. G. Marko guided her out of the port of Novorossisk, she was fatally struck on the starboard side by the Soviet bulk carrier *Pyotr Vasev* and sunk for a second time, with a loss of 423 lives.

Given the *Nakhimov/Berlin* tragedy, and the earlier *Nakhimov* cruiser debacle, it is beyond comprehension why Russian navy brass, in 1992, would decide to rename one of their modern *Kirov*-class heavy missile cruisers—a nuclear-powered ship that had been named *Kalinin* when launched—as *Admiral Nakhimov*. Sailors serving aboard this missile cruiser who knew the fate of the two previous unlucky ships with the same name must have wondered at their superiors' rationale in creating yet another *Admiral Nakhimov*. Was it not just a tad incautious to use that name again, especially on a vessel powered by a nuclear reactor?

At last report the nuclear-powered cruiser is still afloat. But while researching this story in December 2003, the author by chance discovered some additional "real time" news in the Russian media. The daily newspaper *Pravda* reported that on December 2 at 7:23 AM Moscow time, a Russian tugboat sank in the Sea of Azov (a body of water connected by the Kerch Strait to the Black Sea), not far from Sevastopol where Admiral Pavel Stepanovich Nakhimov had won acclaim almost 150 years before. The name painted on the wheelhouse of the unfortunate tug? *Admiral Nakhimov,* of course!

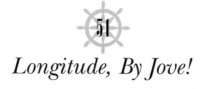

Longitude, By Jove!

L ong before clock maker John Harrison perfected a chronometer sufficiently accurate to be invaluable to mariners in determining longitude at sea, learned scholars had made a number of attempts to find longitude using nature's universal timepiece—the daily parade of celestial objects including the sun, moon, and stars across the sky.

By 1610 Pisa-born genius Galileo Galilei had perfected an earlier Dutch optical invention known as the refracting telescope. Galileo's refinement of this long-distance viewing instrument, and the celestial wonders he uncovered using it, eventually earned for him a guest appearance before the Catholic Inquisition and a bit of jail time, but not before he observed the heavens in more detail than had ever before been possible. Galileo saw for the first time sunspots and the cratered surface of the earth's moon; he took special note of the planet Jupiter and four previously unknown bodies orbiting it—the captive moons Io, Callisto, Europa, and Ganymede.

Galileo recorded eclipses and periods of the Jovian moons, eventually concluding that their regular clockwise motions about the mother planet might be of particular value to seamen attempting to discover their longitude at sea. Astronomers quickly hailed Galileo's much-improved telescope, but his idea for using the movements of Jupiter's satellites to find longitude at sea was unfortunately shelved for the next 150 years.

Interestingly, it was a British churchman and astronomer, Dr. Nevil Maskelyne (the gentleman responsible for the first *Nautical Almanac* in 1767), who resurrected Galileo's navigational idea. Maskelyne attacked John Harrison's attempts to create an accurate mechanical timepiece for navigators as not worthy of serious consideration, especially since the Creator had already so thoughtfully set in motion the master clockwork of Jupiter's satellites. While he was an intelligent and gifted scholar, Maskelyne was no sailor. He failed to appreciate the impracticality of aiming and keeping a three-foot telescope trained on Jupiter in anything but a flat calm sea. When that tiny flaw was pointed out to him, he designed a gimbaled "marine chair" for shipboard observations, which was supposed to allow the observer and telescope to remain horizontally stable in much the same way a gimbaled ship's compass negotiates the yawing, pitching, and rolling motions of a vessel at sea. The chair and its motions instead succeeded only in making the seated observer violently ill. The chair was a total failure and perhaps a bit ahead of its time, if one considers it would have made a great amusement park ride.

As elegant and appealing as scientists and astronomers found this idea for solving the age-old problem of discovering longitude at sea, the true value of the exercise was to be found ashore. Captain James Cook used Jovian moon observations to find Greenwich time and determined his longitude on various coasts during a round-the-world voyage of exploration, making his observations on solid, newfound terra firma. A special navigational benefit of Cook's land-based observations was that he had an accurate point of departure from which to begin the next leg of his voyage.

The New Practical Navigator (the nineteenth edition, published by John Hamilton Moore in 1814) offered navigators the following detailed, if somewhat confusing, instructions for determining longitude accurately using observations of eclipses of Jupiter's moons:

> On the day preceding the evening on which it is proposed to observe an eclipse, look for the time when it will happen at Greenwich, in page 3d of the month in the Ephemeris. Find the difference of longitude either by a good map, sea chart, or dead reckoning. Let the watch be regulated by the sun with all possible exactness to the apparent time. Turn the difference of longitude into time, according as it is east or west of Greenwich, the sum or difference will be nearly the time when the eclipse is to be looked for in that place. But as the longitude is uncertain, it will be proper to begin 20 or 30 minutes before. Observe the hours, minutes, and seconds of the beginning of the eclipse, called immersion, that is, the very instant that the satellite appears to enter the shadow of Jupiter; or the emersion, that is, when it appears to come out of the same. The difference of time between the observed immersion, or emersion, and that set

down in the *Nautical Almanack*, being turned into degrees, will give the difference of longitude between Greenwich and the place of observation.

While the *Nautical Almanac and Astronomical Ephemeris* for many years continued to offer detailed information on the eclipses of Jupiter's moons, sailors rarely practiced this method for finding longitude at sea. Less expensive and more accurate knockoffs of John Harrison's ingenious marine chronometer made certain of that.

The First Lighter-than-Aircraft Carrier

Thaddeus Lowe had always enjoyed getting high as a youth. Lowe had little formal education, but he fancied a career as an "aeronaut," or balloon pilot, from his earliest years. His later theories on air currents and balloon travel led him to believe he could navigate a balloon to any geographic point simply by choosing the appropriate altitude where the wind blew in the direction he desired to travel.

After a number of successful ascents in a balloon of his own construction, he undertook an air voyage on April 20, 1861, from Cincinnati, Ohio, to test his theories.

As with many geniuses, Lowe paid little attention to the momentous political events unfolding around him. When his craft landed in a field near the border between North and South Carolina, some nine hundred miles from Cincinnati, he was quickly introduced to the latest political upheaval, the Civil War. Lowe was immediately surrounded by a mob who thought him a Union spy. Fortunately for Lowe, local authorities arrested him before the mob could demonstrate to him their method for getting Yankee aeronauts airborne—lynching.

When finally released by his captors, Lowe decided to investigate the military possibilities of ballooning. In Washington that June, he demonstrated a reconnaissance balloon to President Lincoln and assorted military brass. Ever the showman, Lowe sent a telegraph message from the balloon's gondola to the surprised president.

Lincoln, visibly impressed, appointed Lowe to the position of Aeronautics Corps chief and head of production and operation of military observation balloons. As chief aeronaut, Lowe soon met John A. Dahlgren, commander of the Washington Navy Yard and another born genius—Dahlgren had designed the famous Dahlgren gun, which revolutionized warfare a decade earlier and would be the cause of much bloodshed on both sides during the unfolding war.

With navy funds, Dahlgren and Lowe obtained and modified an eighty-by-fifteen-foot coal barge to accommodate an onboard reconnaissance balloon, a hangar, winches, and a self-contained gas-generating plant for producing hydrogen gas from iron filings and sulfuric acid. The resulting balloon carrier, christened *George Washington Parke Custis*, became the United States' first true aircraft carrier (or maybe that should be lighter-than-aircraft carrier).

On November 11, 1861, the sophisticated vessel was towed to a tributary of the Potomac River. The balloon was inflated with gas and slowly winched out to its thousand-foot operational ceiling to begin observing and reporting on Confederate troop movements just three miles away. By war's end the hydrogen-filled observation balloon had executed numerous safe ascents, suggesting that Lowe and his assistants were most likely all nonsmokers.

Unfortunately for marine aviation, Lowe lost interest in ballooning after the war and became passionately involved with new scientific interests, including the production of artificial ice and construction of an inclined railway on a mountain in California. *George Washington Parke Custis* was decommissioned and returned to mundane coal-carrying duties.

It should be noted that earlier, on August 3, 1861, balloonist John LaMountain made military observations from a hot-air balloon launched from USS *Fanny*. But *Fanny* performed other naval war duties and was not used exclusively as a launching platform for the balloon. Because *George Washington Parke Custis* was modified and employed exclusively as a balloon-launching vessel, it retains the title of being America's first aircraft carrier.

53

Strange Marine Chronometers

Glass is a "rigid liquid" commonly made up of silica sand, soda ash, lime, and sodium nitrate. Its relative cheapness to produce and resistance to corrosion in the marine environment led the chronometer firm of Arnold and Dent, Number 50 The Strand, London, to undertake various experiments during the early 1830s to study the suitability of using glass in the manufacture of balance springs for marine chronometers.

For sixty years the chronometer had been in use at sea to aid the navigator in accurately determining his longitude. But even after six decades of development and refinement, this special navigational clock was still prohibitively expensive and beyond the reach of the average shipmaster, who relied instead on the cumbersome and often inaccurate "lunar distance" method of observation to find his position east or west of the Meridian of Greenwich.

Arnold and Dent believed that the balance springs they developed of specially formulated glass could offer navigators the possibility of a cheaper chronometer, while having better regulation and greater resistance to corrosion in a salt air environment.

By the middle of 1833 experiments had been completed on the nature and properties of the glass required to produce a functional balance spring. A series of tests were then initiated to study the expansive tendency of glass as temperature increases in comparison with metals.

Arnold and Dent began thermal testing of the glass balance spring by first installing a special glass spring, made "in house," in a used and adjusted chronometer. The chronometer was heated in a controlled environment and the rate results recorded. This test revealed that the chronometer had been overcompensated for temperature changes. They then investigated what error differences might be found in a controlled change-of-temperature test using springs made of gold, steel, and glass.

They selected three identical, used, and adjusted chronometers of conventional construction. The compensation balance was removed from each chronometer and replaced with a plain glass disk with either a gold, steel, or glass balance spring installed. They assumed no errors would arise from the balances, except those generated by changes in air temperature.

The three uncompensated chronometers were collectively exposed in a chamber to an air temperature of thirty degrees Fahrenheit. Over an unknown period of time the temperature was slowly raised in the chamber until it reached one hundred degrees F. The experiment revealed that the chronometer with the gold balance spring fared worst, losing eight minutes and four seconds over the duration of the test. The chronometer with the steel balance spring did somewhat better, losing a total of six minutes and eight seconds during the test period. The chronometer with glass spring lost only forty seconds during the test, much better than the gold and steel springs. The test again suggested that a glass balance spring would require little temperature compensation compared with those of steel or gold composition.

With these test results, Arnold and Dent felt justified in preparing an adjusted chronometer equipped with a glass balance spring in late 1833. In fact two were prepared, the first by order of the Lords of the Admiralty for testing at sea by the Royal Navy. This timekeeper was entrusted to Captain William Hewette of HMS *Fairy*, to be tried during survey work. Unfortunately, HMS *Fairy* was later lost in a vicious storm while surveying in the North Sea. The second chronometer, Number 616, was delivered to the Astronomer Royal at Greenwich Observatory and testing began on January 1, 1834. Although it was not entered into competition with other chronometers in the 1834 chronometer accuracy trials, Number 616 was placed in the same testing room with trial chronometers from other makers and with three timekeepers of conventional design by Arnold and Dent. Here it was exposed to the same temperature variations as the trial chronometers, but was not eligible for the prizes offered for extreme accuracy in timekeeping. The trial that year had twenty-eight chronometers entered; Number 616's rate of 2.72 seconds would have been good enough for a second-place prize had it been entered in the competition.

For some unexplained reason glass balance springs seem not to have been employed in later chronometer construction, despite their proven usefulness in imparting great accuracy to the timepieces in which they were installed. The glass balance spring of the chronometer installed aboard HMS *Fairy* may have failed sea tests before *Fairy* was lost, or it may have gone to the bottom in perfectly good order. For whatever reason, further sea testing of glass balance springs seems not to have been undertaken by the famous chronometer makers Arnold and Dent—their reason for halting further development of the innovative springs now lost amid the detritus of marine horological history.

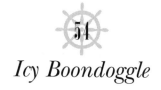

Icy Boondoggle

One of the more bizarre areas of marine research in England during World War II concerned proposed development of a very unusual kind of war vessel.

In 1942 the only way to get both fighter and bomber aircraft from America to beleaguered England was to transport them by ship; they could not be flown that distance given fuel volume limitations. Germany's U-boats had mastered the Atlantic, and the loss of shipping tonnage to torpedoes was staggering. To overcome the problem of getting aircraft to Britain, the Admiralty and Prime Minister Winston Churchill were willing to consider any idea, no matter how bizarre.

One such idea that crossed the desks of the Admiralty and the prime minister involved human-made icebergs—more specifically, a fleet of unsinkable icebergs that could be stationed at various points across the Atlantic as landing fields and refueling depots for aircraft being ferried to England. The bergs would be towed from Arctic waters and armored around the edges in some way to protect them from submarine attack.

The British Admiralty's specs for the bergs required that they should be at least four thousand feet long to accommodate landing strips for larger aircraft, be maneuverable using propellers driven by electric motors, and be capable of continuing to function even if struck constantly by torpedoes or mines—a sort of frosty aircraft carrier. British economic advisers suggested that the large number of torpedoes that would be necessary to inflict even a small amount of damage to one of these icy landing fields would—at twenty-five thousand German marks a pop—bring economic instability to German banks funding the Nazi war effort.

While other top-secret, high-profile projects were carefully hidden away from prying enemy eyes in both Manhattan and Peenemunde, Germany, this outrageous scheme called London its home. It was housed beneath a butcher shop, presumably because refrigeration equipment was available. A research laboratory was soon established to work on technical aspects of armoring ice. In five underground floors of the commandeered property, Dr. Max Ferdinand Perutz and his colleagues worked in freezing conditions, wearing protective, electrically heated lab suits, experimenting with various ice "cocktails" to produce a kind of ice cement called Pykrete, after one of the project's advisers, Geoffrey Pyke.

At a time when the United States and Germany worked on the "ridiculous" ideas of nuclear weapons and ballistic missiles, Britain forged ahead with the much more sensible iceberg "weapon." Pyke even foresaw specially prepared icebergs being deployed as super siege platforms with which to attack Japan and invade France.

The project, which might have made an ideal story for a Marvel Comics issue, finally melted away after the flying range of aircraft being sent to England had been increased sufficiently to allow them to be flown directly to England, without the necessity of refueling en route.

It is interesting to speculate how German submarine wolf packs might have tactically dealt with any "HMS *Iceberg*" they might discover in mid-Atlantic. Perhaps the U-boats would have attacked the floating airfields in more unconventional ways, approaching their enemy on the surface, having removed their eighty-eight-millimeter deck cannons and substituted in their place—giant hair dryers with which to melt the enemy vessels.

55

Lightning Strikes Again

Contemporary sailors of sailing vessels often give little thought to their boat's lightning-protection system until they see the flashes of an approaching storm. Few know that they owe their safety to a little-known investigator named W. T. Harris. Harris looked long and carefully at the dreadful effects of lightning strikes at sea in the nineteenth century before developing a scientific theory, and then a physical solution for control of this phenomenon aboard ship.

Early sailors often carried amulets and charms to protect them from whichever god happened to be tossing fiery bolts in their direction. An old engraving shows a dripping Viking warrior standing high in the bow of his longship in a violent sea gale, lightning flashing above in the heavens and he, raising his great double-edged sword high in defiance of the thunder god Thor. Needless to say, some of these early protection methods proved somewhat more hazardous than others.

Harris began serious investigations into the nature of lightning phenomena by studying the writings of earlier natural philosophers, including Ben Franklin, who proposed the use of lightning rods on buildings to safely lead the "electric fluid" to the ground during storms. He also studied the effects of strikes on hundreds of vessels such as the American ship *Amphion*, bound for Rio de Janeiro in 1822. *Amphion* received a lightning strike on her mizzenmast, destroying her compasses, bulkheads, and rudder trunk as well as most of her cabin furniture, before passing out through the quarterdeck into the sea. The Royal Navy's ninety-gun HMS *Duke* was similarly struck by a bolt at the island of Martinique in 1793, while she was engaging an enemy shore battery. *Duke* suffered heavy damage, including the disintegration of her maintopmast—not to mention severe damage to the crew's morale when they witnessed what appeared to be the intervention of heaven itself on behalf of the enemy. During the attack on Havana in 1762 by British and colonial American forces, an armed Spanish merchantman anchored in

Havana Harbor was similarly struck by lightning and destroyed when her powder magazine exploded while the battle raged.

Harris successfully asked and answered the question of "how far it is possible to parry the violent operation of discharges on shipboard." He proposed to "perfect the conducting power of the masts . . . together with that of the rigging . . . by efficient copper conductors," which would then be connected by copper wires to copper sheets on the bottom of the vessel. He further proposed to "connect in a similar way, all the detached metal bodies of the ship, both with each other and the general system" to complete "the conducting power of the whole mass, and remove all resistance to the process of electrical diffusion."

Estimates for installing Harris's ingenious lightning-protection system on a First Rate naval ship of 120 guns were £60 for labor and £306 for copper sheeting and wire. While this was a considerable sum at the time, it seemed money well spent to protect a man-of-war that, when fully equipped, could be worth as much as £110,000. Even today, the protection afforded by a well-installed boat grounding system based on the ideas of Harris justifies the expense involved.

56

In the Eye of the Beholder

Back in Royalist France of 1762, Monsieur Etienne Bottineau was a minor cog in the great bureaucratic clockwork that was the navy of Louis XVI. Born in the Loire River Valley about 1740, Bottineau was destined to develop what could only be described as a truly visionary idea, one that would later allow him to baffle his peers and a senior political functionary with his inexplicable ability to predict with great precision the arrival times of inbound ships to ports—achieving this feat well before those ships' topsails could be spotted coming over the horizon, apparently only by watching for special signs that he perceived in the atmosphere.

Bottineau theorized that a vessel approaching a coast should produce some kind of physical change in the coastal atmosphere that would reveal the vessel's near proximity to anyone who had honed the special visual skills necessary for observing the effect. The young sailor's first attempts discouraged him, as he was correct in predicting the approach of a vessel only about half the time—a record that disheartened him so much that he almost decided to give up practicing and refining his observational technique.

In 1767, while he was still experimenting with his pet theory, Bottineau accepted a post at the isolated French colony of Ile de France (now Mauritius), east of Madagascar in the Indian Ocean. King Louis's government had taken over control of Ile de France from the French East India Company, and Bottineau was to play a small part within the island's new administrative structure.

Being posted to Port Louis, the capital of Ile de France, must have been rather like being sentenced today to a tour of duty at the South Pole, only with warm breezes and palm trees. But Bottineau's remote situation apparently suited him just fine, since the new posting would allow him ample free time to experiment with his theory in a climate where fine, clear weather most days was the norm. After six months on the island Bottineau was sure he had perfected his method—he was now getting much better results with his predictions of vessel arrivals. He coined the term *Nauscopy* to describe his odd nautical theory.

Most naval and military officers on the island led idle, sedentary lives of card playing, drinking, or (if really motivated) strolling along the shore with telescopes, watching for vessels arriving from Europe. Bottineau frequently laid wagers with these bored fellow exiles that a vessel would arrive at a given time in the future, sometimes as much as four days before she would actually be spotted by the "vigies," or coast lookouts. He was now rarely wrong in his predictions and soon amassed a tidy sum of money through his betting. The officers were puzzled by Bottineau's uncanny ability, since he used no telescope, nor any other instrument, in making his predictions—only his eyes. Some of the more superstitious among them called him a wizard—a dabbler in the black arts. Eventually no one would accept his bets.

In 1780 Bottineau finally decided to announce his discovery to France's newly appointed senior naval official, Charles de Castries, *le ministre de marine*, in the hope that he might sell his matured idea for a significant sum of government cash. De Castries did read Bottineau's letter but was skeptical of his claims. However, he decided to contact the governor of Ile de France, François le Vicomte de Souillac, instructing him to begin keeping a detailed record of all of Bottineau's predictions for the next two years, just to see if the man's crazy claims had any merit. Thus a controlled series of observations was begun on May 15, 1782. The second day Bottineau reported to De Souillac that three vessels were nearing the island. Orders were then given to the port vigies to carefully scan the horizon for the first sign of any vessels. They reported none, but on May 17 one lookout reported that the topsails of a vessel had just appeared over the horizon. On the eighteenth, a second ship came into sight, followed on the twenty-sixth by a third vessel. At this point De Souillac, who was convinced of Bottineau's skills by his many earlier successes, took it upon himself to offer Bottineau ten thousand livres (about one hundred thousand present-day US dollars) on behalf of the French government and a further yearly pension of twelve hundred livres a year to reveal his secret. Bottineau declined the offer, believing he could do much better if he could just get back to France to demonstrate his technique to De Castries personally.

De Souillac, in a letter to De Castries, vouched for Bottineau's authenticity, reporting that he truly believed the man had discovered a valuable nautical skill that could reliably predict the presence of vessels as far as two hundred leagues at sea using nothing more than his eyes. De Souillac also related an earlier incident when Bottineau predicted a fleet of eleven vessels was approaching the island—a bit of news that threw the entire French garrison of Port Louis into alarm, in fear it might be a force of Royal Navy ships with orders to attack. A fast sloop was sent to shadow the supposed British fleet, but before it returned with any news, Bottineau reported to the governor that the signs he had spotted in the sky had disappeared—an event that he said meant the ships had altered course away from the island. Shortly afterward a French East India vessel entered port, her captain reporting that he had barely managed to evade a powerful fleet of British vessels. This event may have solidified the governor's faith in Bottineau's skill and demonstrated to him the possible military value of Nauscopy.

De Souillac's letter also recounted that for a four-year period beginning in 1778 Bottineau had correctly and publicly announced the arrival of 575 inbound vessels, a large number of those as many as four days before they became visible to the island's lookouts, using telescopes. De Souillac assured De Castries that Bottineau could not be an impostor because of these many proven successes in prediction.

The letter written by De Souillac probably did reach De Castries's offices, but his secretaries may never have brought it to his attention, as De Souillac appears never to have received a reply. In the meantime, a frustrated Bottineau decided to catch a lift back home to France aboard one of King Louis's ships in 1784. During the voyage he entertained a curious Captain Dufour and his crew by correctly predicting the approach of twenty-seven ships. As the voyage continued around southern Africa, Bottineau was surprised to discover that he was also capable of foreseeing his own ship's approach to land in a way similar to his "seeing" approaching vessels. On one occasion he informed Dufour that his ship was not more than thirty leagues from land. Dufour argued that this was impossible, but since the captain had seen Bottineau's skills well demonstrated, he decided to recheck his navigational calculations. Upon reexamining his reckoning he found an error, altered course, and apologized to Bottineau. Bottineau successfully found land three times on the voyage, once at a distance of 150 leagues (about 450 nautical miles).

When he arrived in Paris, Bottineau's persistent attempts to see the very busy De Castries were thwarted by the minister's assistants, possibly because De Castries had been honored by the king with the additional title of *marechal de France* in 1783, giving him increased responsibilities and putting his valuable time at a premium. Bottineau was similarly frustrated in trying to find a respected scientist to investigate his theory. He went to local newspapers with his story. Most laughed at his ideas, with the editor of the *Mercure de France* being particularly malicious in an editorial in which he mocked Bottineau's theories. By this time the first clouds of political unease were drifting across France, heralding the preamble to the French Revolution. The scientific minds of the period may have been too preoccupied with the changing political mood in France to invest time in a detailed scientific investigation of Bottineau's theory of Nauscopy, or they may have discounted the theory out of hand, without further reflection.

A discouraged Etienne Bottineau, developer of the still-unproved science he called Nauscopy, finally returned to Ile de France where his name and skills were still held in some esteem, and where he could at least count on getting a little respect. He died at Port Louis in 1813 without ever having had his theory properly investigated by men of science. Bottineau's Nauscopy might have benefited the advancement of the practice of marine navigation, and possibly contributed to France's becoming the foremost marine power of the world. The only major drawback to Bottineau's theory, if it did prove useful, would seem to be that the practice of Nauscopy would have to be confined to daylight hours only.

POSTSCRIPT

Bottineau defined *Nauscopy* as "the art of ascertaining the approach of vessels, or, being in a vessel, the approach to land, at a very great distance." When a vessel approaches land, or another vessel, a phenomenon that he called a meteor became visible to him. A historical dictionary reference for the eighteenth century says of the term *meteor*:

> Atmospheric phenomena were formerly often classed as aerial or
> airy meteors (winds), aqueous or watery meteors (rain, snow, hail,

dew, etc.), luminous meteors (the aurora, rainbows, halo, etc.), and igneous or fiery meteors (lightning, shooting stars, etc.)

An English translation of Etienne Bottineau's lengthy explanation of Nauscopy was carried in *Nautical Magazine* for March 1834. The author offers this condensed version of the translation for would-be Nauscopists:

As animal and vegetable matter decays in the world's oceans, large volumes of various gases are released into and trapped by seawater. These gases are released only when the water is agitated either by rough weather or by a ship's bow slicing through its surface. The movement of the ship releases some of the trapped gases, which then rise into the air as an invisible cloud of vapor. This vapor cloud surrounds the vessel, advances with it, and increases in size as the vessel moves forward. As the ship continues to sail on its course, one end of the growing vapor cloud remains at the ship while the other end extends forward a significant distance. According to Bottineau, this vapor cloud remains invisible until it encounters vapors rising from land or another vessel. At the point when and where these two vapors meet, a person experienced in the science of Nauscopy will observe subtle changes in the atmosphere, including visible changes in what he called consistence and color tone. Bottineau also stated that stormy weather would not destroy the effect, only delay it somewhat.

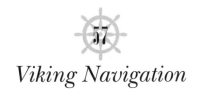

Viking Navigation

In the distance a pall of black smoke rises over a distinctly Monty Pythonesque scene. Houses burn while women scream and run from a marauding horde of sea wolves who have just stormed ashore from their longboats to raid this tenth-century settlement. An Anglo-Saxon peasant, looking suspiciously like John Cleese, frantically flees from a giant, ax-wielding Viking who might be mistaken for the governor of a large US West Coast state. The peasant stumbles, then falls as the burly warrior catches up. The Viking raises his ax to strike the cowering peasant as the peasant blurts out:

> I say, old chap, just how did you manage to navigate your way here from your far northern land, to burn our village and ravage our women?

The Viking chuckles and replies, while raising a brawny arm to bring his ax down upon his hapless victim:

> That's easy, Briton—I just followed the birds.

In fact, it was the observation of the migration patterns of birds that first supplied navigational cues to early Viking seafarers. The first voyages from Scandinavia to Ireland and Scotland were made because their geographic positions were betrayed to the keen-eyed Vikings by seasonal flights of birds between these lands. On longer voyages of exploration to the west, they also noted that any bird joining their boat in mid-ocean would usually stay aboard until flying distance to the nearest land was reached, assuming the bird could avoid falling into the clutches of the longboat's chef. A Viking named Floki (known to his boat buddies as the Raven) routinely carried ravens aboard his longboat to be released at intervals during voyages. If a raven returned to the boat after release,

Floki assumed there was no land nearby. If the raven failed to return, the boat was probably close to land.

The Vikings did have a good motivation for continuously developing their navigational skills between the eighth and eleventh centuries CE. Iceland, Greenland, and finally "Vinland" in the New World were all discovered mainly because the Norse peoples were running out of good farmland at home, and were increasingly unable to support an ever-growing population. Developing their particular navigational skills to search for new lands became an important social necessity.

But they did not, during their first explorations, develop a knowledge of navigation as we understand it today. Theirs was a special form of navigation based on the observation of the nature of their marine environment and the night sky, similar in some respects to that of Polynesian navigators.

Before 1000 CE, Viking sailors had developed a method of defining direction at sea. They observed that each day the sun would climb to a maximum height in the sky before falling again toward the horizon. By watching the shadow of the mast, or some other part of the ship, as the sun moved through its daily arc, they could steer a relatively straight course. The direction of the sun at its highest daily altitude—and the opposite direction—actually defined for them two directional ideas: those of "south" and "north." In addition, since the coasts of Scandinavia run in a mostly north–south direction, the men of the longboats developed the concept of "land" and "outland." That is, directions on the landward side of north or south (northeast or southeast) were called land-north or land-south. Similarly, directions away from the land were called outland-north or outland-south. They also learned to estimate their boat speed and distance traveled by counting oar strokes. It is unlikely that the Vikings used the Pole Star for "latitude sailing" in early discovery voyages, but it did provide them with a steering guide at night, as did the sun during the day. Latitude hooks and lodestone compasses were available only after Iceland, Greenland, and "Vinland" had been discovered.

The sun of course did not always shine in the gloomy northern latitudes, so the Vikings additionally developed quite innovative methods for finding their approximate position using their senses. They could smell the spruce and fir forests of Labrador and their homeland long before they could see them. They also took cues from observing the color of the water, its density, its temperature as measured by dipping a hand over the side, then smelling the water and even tasting it for salinity. Viking navigators who were not as skilled as might be hoped in finding land could expect to be thrown over the side by disgruntled shipmates, to be towed behind so that they might more intimately observe all the data at once, in real time. This would also assist towees in maintaining personal hygiene.

Primitive "sounding-leads" were also used to indicate the approach to land. With tallow attached to the bottom of the lead, northern navigators could identify a particular coast or landfall, even in foggy conditions, by examining the type and color of material that stuck to the tallow. When the lead hit the bottom, the tallow would pick up pebbles, sand, or mud, and the knowledgeable Viking navigator could, by noting the cues offered by the bottom material, make a fairly accurate return to a previously visited coast.

The Vikings were keen observers of eddies and currents, and were especially adept at interpreting interference wave patterns created by the action of winds, currents, and nearby landmasses. They also took navigational cues from watching clouds. Northern navigators observed that clouds tended to line up along coasts, and that clouds often hugged the tops of mountains, making the discovery of land possible long before those same mountains appeared on the horizon. And they almost certainly were acquainted with those unusual sea and sky conditions that resulted in mirages, or reflected images of land below the horizon being made visible. Reflected glare from ice- or snow-covered land gave a similar cue that a newfound land might be waiting just over the horizon.

Dr. R. Robin Baker, author of *Human Navigation and the Sixth Sense*, has conducted extensive experiments in Britain that suggest all human beings have, to some degree, a magnetic sense of direction much like birds'. This sense gradually falls into disuse when terrestrial cues such as mountains, trees, and rocks are available. Is it possible that the Vikings, having spent so much of their lives at sea away from any fixed visual reference, actually relied in part on some rudimentary magnetic "sixth sense" to enhance their unusual navigational prowess? Perhaps only Odin knows for sure.

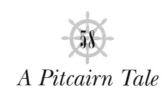

A Pitcairn Tale

S ituated about halfway between South America and Australia (approximately 25 degrees south and 130 degrees east), and barely two
square miles in area, lonely Pitcairn Island conjures up images of the
most celebrated marine mutiny of all time—the mutiny on HMS *Bounty*.

The island was serendipitously discovered in 1766 by the English
navigator Philip Carteret while he was engaged in a circumnavigation of
the globe. Pitcairn takes its name from the sailor aboard Carteret's ship,
Swallow, who was first to spot the tiny island peeping over the horizon.

But Pitcairn owes its true niche in history to events surrounding the
seizure of HMS *Bounty* by part of her crew and to the legendary animos-
ity between *Bounty*'s first mate, Fletcher Christian, and his nemesis, the
infamous Captain William Bligh.

Bligh was an experienced and able enough Royal Navy man, having
spent his early years on three successive vessels before being chosen by
Captain James Cook to act as sailing master for his third voyage of exploration in HMS *Resolution*. But in 1788 Bligh found himself in command of his own ship, *Bounty*, on a voyage to Tahiti. Bligh's orders were
to collect young breadfruit trees at Tahiti, which were to be transported
to the West Indies for evaluation as a possible cheap food source for
plantation slaves.

Fletcher Christian had been handpicked by Bligh to act as first mate
for the voyage, but their good working relationship seems to have slowly
deteriorated as the voyage progressed. Mutual hatred grew to the point
that Christian actually planned to leave the ship on a makeshift raft.
However, some of the crew who knew of his plans convinced him to remain and lead them in a general revolt against Bligh's tyrannical rule.

But Bligh's oppressive leadership style was not the only reason for
the shipboard coup d'état. The crew found the women and the idyllic,
unfettered lifestyle of Tahiti very much more to their liking than the
harsh and cheerless existence offered them in one of His Britannic

Majesty's ships. So, on April 28, 1789, while *Bounty* was off Tofua in the Friendly Islands, Fletcher Christian and his cohorts seized control of the vessel from Bligh and eighteen of the ship's complement who remained loyal to their captain.

Bligh and the faithful eighteen were cast adrift in *Bounty*'s twenty-three-foot launch, with only few provisions and no charts. After a grueling voyage of more than thirty-six hundred nautical miles, fraught with danger and extreme hardship, Bligh and his men finally reached safety at Timor on June 14.

Meanwhile, the mutinous mariners made their way with *Bounty* back to the maidens of Tahiti. Eventually Fletcher Christian and eight of his men decided to leave Tahiti, sailing *Bounty* to isolated Pitcairn Island with six Tahitian men and twelve Tahitian women on board. Christian also had with him the famous and well-traveled chronometer known as K-2 (Larcum Kendall's copy of a John Harrison–designed navigational watch), which Bligh had brought with him on the Tahiti voyage. When *Bounty* arrived at Pitcairn, the mutineers ran the ship aground at the southern end of the island, then proceeded to establish the first permanent settlement. (Remains of HMS *Bounty* were located and identified in 1957.)

When the Admiralty finally learned of the mutiny, HMS *Pandora* was dispatched to round up those mutineers still at Tahiti. Ten men were eventually tried at Portsmouth, England, but only three were actually hanged.

Meanwhile, the settlement on Pitcairn continued without British interference. When the American whaler *Topaz* visited the island in 1809, John Adams was the only mutineer still alive. Adams was the undisputed community leader, and the settlement, Adamstown, had been named in his honor. Adams also had in his possession Kendall's chronometer, which he sold to *Topaz*'s captain. Adams eventually received a full royal pardon for his part in the mutiny, and died in 1829.

As it turned out, the breadfruit tree experiment was a flop. Plantation owners in the West Indies eventually settled on the banana-like plantain plant as the staple of choice for feeding their slaves.

Bligh survived the ordeal only to have the extraordinary honor of being at the center of a second humiliating mutiny in 1808, while he was governor of New South Wales, Australia. Soldiers under his command rebelled against his oppressive authority and threw him in prison. Incredibly, his leadership abilities were still not questioned by the Admiralty. After he was freed his naval career continued; eventually he rose to the rank of vice admiral.

The final destiny of Fletcher Christian remains uncertain. He and three of his men were thought to have been killed on Pitcairn by some of the transplanted Tahitians in 1794. There have also been suggestions that he escaped the island and returned to England in secret. The true account of what happened to Christian will probably never be known, as John Adams took that secret with him to the grave.

59

Penny-Pinching Purser

Whether he was serving in the fledgling Republican Navy of the United States or the Royal Navy of King George III, the purser exercised a powerful influence on the lives of all aboard naval vessels at the end of the eighteenth century.

Entrusted with provisioning vessels of war, the "pusser"—as he was more commonly known—was also the butt of jokes among ship's crew for being a miserly and often dishonest seller of clothing and tobacco in the pre-uniform navies of the United States and Great Britain.

The purser frequently became a wealthy man at the expense of his government and ship's company. He had several sources of income. First, he received a small salary from his officer's commission in the navy; second and more lucrative was a commission on the issuing of the daily victualing allowance of the ship. He drew from stores at sixteen ounces to the pound and provided the ship's needs at fourteen ounces to the pound, giving him a two-ounce profit on every food stock he measured out. This fourteen-ounce pound became known as the "pusser's pound."

The purser lived a decidedly lonely life in a bureaucratic world of warrants, receipts, and records. He was responsible for safe stowage and constant inspection of ship's stores, especially liquid stores in casks. A leaking beer cask, for instance, could become a bureaucratic nightmare. The event was handled thusly: The captain first had to issue a "warrant" to the master and two additional officers of the ship, who were to provide in writing, on the back of the warrant, an assessment of the quantity of beer or other valuable liquid store lost, as well as the reason for its leakage. The ship's cooper also had to give an "oath" as to the condition of the leaking container. Seamen were often in the habit of drilling small holes in stored casks so that they could obtain a clandestine drink with the aid of a piece of straw.

An additional source of income for the purser was the "slop chest." Slops (from the Old English *sloppe*, meaning "breeches") were ready-made articles of clothing for sale to the crew, usually of poor-quality material and manufacture, and purchased from cheap sources ashore by the purser. In the days before issuance of uniforms in both the US and Royal Navies, this was the only source of clothing for the seamen. As their slowly rotting clothes began to fall off, the crew were forced to purchase, against their next pay, overpriced, thin, and ill-fitting clothes from the purser when he next opened his slop chest (on specified days of the month).

The purser also had the right to sell tobacco to the crew at appointed times, but was restricted (at least in the Royal Navy) to selling two pounds per month to each man—another of his lucrative sources of income. No wonder then that the crew often hated the man who was the only shipboard source of basic personal needs at exorbitant prices.

When he quit the navy, the purser often took his considerable savings and skimmings and opened a tavern or inn ashore, one of the few lower-ranking naval men who could expect to end his days in more-than-comfortable circumstances.

60

Troop Queen

W hat could a stockman from New South Wales, a stockbroker from New York, and a railway telegrapher from Nova Scotia possibly have in common? Between 1942 and 1944 they, and thousands of their countrymen, were military "guests" aboard the fastest and most modern ocean liner afloat, the Cunard-owned RMS *Queen Elizabeth.*

The 82,998-ton *Queen Elizabeth* was modified for troop transport, and her designation RMS (Royal Mail Ship) was dropped for HMT (His Majesty's Transport) for the duration of World War II. During that time she carried nearly half of all Allied troops sent to Europe. *Queen Elizabeth* was a true behemoth, capable of carrying sixteen thousand troops per trip (on one voyage she transported the entire First US Infantry Division) at a speed of more than thirty knots—fast enough that senior naval men felt she could safely avoid the German U-boat fleet of Grand Admiral Karl Donitz.

In salons where one should have found fashionable women in diamonds gossiping about Wallis Simpson and gentlemen lounging with brandies and cigars, only military personnel in fatigues could be found, sitting on jury-rigged bunks often stacked thirty high. The men spent their time sleeping, playing craps, or writhing with paroxysms of seasickness. To relieve the boredom and tension, military men were encouraged to "volunteer" for shipboard duty, filling the jobs of lookout, gun crew, mess orderly, and kitchen helper.

Meals were served only twice each day, in shifts—breakfast from 6:30 to 11 AM and "tea" from 3 to 7:30 PM. While food was adequate and plentiful, it was definitely not of the gourmet variety one might expect to be laid before a passenger aboard this elegant vessel in peacetime. But a sense of decorum was not completely absent—officers were expected to appear in shirt, tie, and jacket for meals, and special holiday dinners were announced on attractive menus printed in the ship's print shop. Following is just part of the provisions stored aboard for one Atlantic crossing:

76,000 pounds of flour and cereals

21,500 pounds of bacon and ham

155,000 pounds of meat and poultry

18,000 pounds of canned jams

31,000 pounds of various canned goods

29,000 pounds of fresh fruit

31,000 pounds of coffee, sugar, and tea

53,600 pounds of butter, eggs, and milk powder

124,300 pounds of potatoes

At one point, Adolf Hitler offered a bounty equivalent to almost $250,000 and an Iron Cross to any Kriegsmarine commander who could send the famous *Queen* to the bottom of the Atlantic. On November 9, 1942, Kapitanleutnant Kessler of *U-704* could hardly contain his glee as he spotted the ultimate prize near fifty-five degrees north, twenty-nine degrees west. No doubt with visions of a comfortable retirement on a Bavarian estate in mind, Kessler cried *"Losen"* and *U-704* released a spread of four torpedoes at the rapidly moving target. The U-boat's crew heard one explosion as the *Queen* slipped into the mist, and Kessler eagerly radioed his handlers that he had a confirmed hit. Unfortunately for Kessler, what he'd heard was one of the torpedoes self-destructing short of its target. *Queen Elizabeth* continued on unharmed, her crew blissfully unaware of the botched attack.

At least one 1944 trip on the *Queen Elizabeth* was considerably more enjoyable for shipboard guests. Glenn Miller's band was aboard, and the main salon echoed with the strains of "In the Mood" and "Moonlight Serenade," making this passage to embattled Britain just a bit more pleasurable than most.

POSTSCRIPT

My father, John James Dill, was the railway telegrapher mentioned at the beginning of this story. In 1942, as a radio operator with the Royal Canadian Corps of Signals, Signalman Dill made a voyage from Halifax to England in HMT *Queen Elizabeth* to begin a tour of duty in England and later Europe.

61

Pirates Attack Mexican

On September 20, 1832, the Salem, Massachusetts, brig *Mexican*, under the command of Captain Butman and bound for Rio de Janeiro in latitude thirty-three degrees north and longitude thirty-four degrees west, found herself under attack by a pirate schooner flying a Brazilian flag.

In short order *Mexican* was boarded and her crew subdued and locked below. The pirates took twenty thousand dollars in cash and everything else of value they could find aboard. Their plunder complete, the pirates set *Mexican* afire, intending to destroy the vessel and her crew to keep their crime from being discovered.

After the schooner bore off, Captain Butman and his crew regained their freedom by escaping through a scuttle, which the pirates had failed to secure. The crew worked feverishly to keep the fire from spreading and with great effort succeeded in putting out the flames. The tired crew then sailed their damaged vessel back to her home port of Salem, Massachusetts. Although the US government ordered a vessel to cruise in pursuit of the pirate schooner, the chase was soon given up as hopeless.

Unknown to the citizens of Salem, their old enemy from the War of 1812, the Royal Navy—specifically HMS *Curlew*—was at that moment in pursuit of the same pirate vessel that had raided *Mexican*, off the coast of Africa. After a short chase the British cruiser had destroyed the pirate schooner, killing or capturing all her crew.

In an unusual move, the British Admiralty decided to transport, at its own expense, the fourteen surviving pirates to the authorities at Salem for trial. This was no doubt done to court the goodwill of a town that had suffered economic hardships under Royal Navy policy, including impressment and seizure of merchant vessels, during the War of 1812. In due course the Admiralty dispatched the criminals aboard the armed brig *Savage* under the command of Lieutenant R. Loney. The citizens of the town received with great courtesy and honor HMS *Savage* and her crew. The *Salem Gazette* reported:

> It is honourable to modern nations that, instead of being asylums of foreign criminals, that the society exists which aids each other in bringing felons to justice . . .

The company that had insured *Mexican* rewarded Lieutenant Loney and the *Savage* crew with a generous supply of quality provisions before they left Salem.

There is no indication what fate befell the pirates. However, it is unlikely the judge recommended that they perform community service to atone for their crimes.

62

Narrow Escape for Rebel Steamer

Near the end of the American Civil War, the Union navy had so effectively blockaded the ports of the Confederacy that trade through them had become virtually strangled. Only a few small, fast vessels were able to run the blockade successfully, sailing primarily from the British colonial ports of Halifax, Nova Scotia; Hamilton, Bermuda; Nassau, Bahamas; and Kingston, Jamaica—all ports having a strong Royal Navy presence.

While Great Britain was officially neutral in the US conflict, factions within the empire were often at odds with the policy of neutrality. So it was not surprising that while Queen Victoria asked for divine support of Mr. Lincoln's moral cause in her nightly prayers, officers of Her Majesty's Royal Navy were frequently aiding the Confederate cause at sea whenever the opportunity presented itself. One of those opportunities came in the early-morning hours of August 21, 1864, when the Confederate cruiser *Tallahassee* slipped into the harbor of "neutral" Halifax, short of coal and provisions, and with US cruisers in pursuit just a few hours behind.

Tallahassee was an impressive ship measured by anyone's standards and a thoroughly modern vessel for her time. She had a sleek, 220-foot, iron-built hull with a 24-foot beam that displaced nearly seven hundred tons. If that was not enough to turn the heads of marine aficionados, her propulsion system would. Belowdecks, directly under her raked twin stacks, sat two coal-fired steam engines capable of developing a total of two hundred horsepower. Coupling that power to twin screws gave *Tallahassee* the ability to make the incredible pursuit speed of seventeen knots and virtually turn on a dime. Built in Britain in 1864, she was originally christened *Atlanta*, and she began her sea career as a blockade-runner making clandestine supply runs between Wilmington and Hamilton in economic support of the Confederacy's cause. Her success at avoiding blockading Union vessels caught the notice of the Confederate government and an experienced military man, John Taylor Wood. In July 1864 the Confederacy purchased *Atlanta* and quickly converted her to serve a new role—that of a commerce raider. She received three heavy guns and a new name, CSS *Tallahassee*. *Tallahassee*'s new commander would be Lieutenant John Taylor Wood.

The pairing of John Wood with *Tallahassee* would be, as time would prove, one of those rare fortunate matches of a determined, daring commander and a fast, well-armed, capable ship. Wood's background was impressive. His grandfather, Zachary Taylor, had been the twelfth president of the United States. His uncle, Jefferson Davis, was president of the Confederate States of America. When he graduated from the US Naval Academy in 1853, he finished second in his class. He served with the US Navy, gaining sea experience during the Mexican War. But with the secession of the South in 1861, Wood's sympathies for the Confederate cause prompted his resignation from the US Navy.

As a seasoned sailor and loyal Southerner, Wood was more than a little aware of the severe damage the blockade of the Confederacy's ports was doing to the economy of the South in 1864. He intended to deliver an equally devastating blow to the economy of the North. To that end *Tallahassee* quietly slipped her moorings at Wilmington Harbor on August 21, 1864, successfully evading blockading vessels under cover of darkness.

Tallahassee and Wood were phenomenally successful in carrying out the plan. In just twenty-one days of cruising the raider had run down and destroyed more than thirty Union merchant vessels between New York and southwestern Nova Scotia. When news of *Tallahassee*'s rampage on the Atlantic coast reached the ears of the secretary of the navy, thirteen armed cruisers were ordered to sea to hunt down the Rebel steamer. By this time Wood was running short of coal and provisions, and her nearest nonhostile port was Halifax. When *Tallahassee* entered Halifax Harbor, three Union ships were in pursuit. The US vessels held back at the harbor's three-mile bell buoy, awaiting the exit of the Confederate cruiser.

Under neutrality provisions, Wood was entitled to remain in port only twenty-four hours—long enough to coal and water his ship. On August 22, 1864, the *Nova Scotian* newspaper gave the following account of a mysterious ship that had entered the harbor the day before:

Yesterday morning, a considerable flutter was created in the community by the appearance of a strange vessel of rakish appearance at the Market Wharf. On inspection the visitor proved to be the Confederate cruiser, the Tallahassee, which had within a short space of twelve days made expensive havoc among Federal merchant vessels off Sandy Hook, New York; Portland, Maine; and in the vicinity of Cape Sable. The Tallahassee is an iron steamer of about 500 tons burthen, and has a powerful engine, and is furnished with two screws, and is the swiftest ocean steamship in the Confederate services, being capable under heavy pressure and steam of making from eighteen to twenty miles per hour. Her sides and smoke stacks are painted white and her bottom red. She carries two formidable swivel guns, one at the bow and another at the stern, and a piece of brass ordnance of smaller calibre forward of her fore mast.

Predictably, Halifax naval personnel made little effort to hide their support for the Confederacy by assisting Wood—this at a time when many prominent Halifax families had sons serving as officers in Maine and Massachusetts regiments. Wood entertained curious RN officers in Southern gentlemanly style, serving glasses of bourbon and proffering cigars while leading his guests on a tour of his modern vessel, which included showing off his extensive and newly acquired collection of trophy chronometers—timely souvenirs removed from US merchant ships before he dispatched them to the bottom of the Atlantic.

When the US consul at Halifax, Mortimer Jackson, got wind of *Tallahassee*'s presence in the harbor, he lost little time in firing off a telegram to the US secretary of the navy, informing him of the presence in this British port of the notorious Confederate ship. Then he banged on the door of the senior British admiral of the port to protest. Admiral Sir James Hope, in predictable Royal Navy fashion, wanted nothing to do with the exasperated Yankee functionary and quickly showed Jackson the door. Undaunted, Jackson drove his carriage the few blocks to the residence of the lieutenant governor of the province, whom he knew had a son fighting with a Massachusetts regiment. Jackson pleaded with the lieutenant governor to forbid the coaling of *Tallahassee*, but to no avail. While the governor's sympathies lay with the Northern cause, he was unable to interfere in a purely naval matter.

With repairs completed, Wood hired Jock Fleming, a local fisherman and sailor with exceptional coastal piloting skills, to guide the Rebel cruiser through the little-used and dangerous eastern passage of Halifax Harbor, at night. Fleming's home was on the shores near the end of the passage, and he knew the narrow route like the back of his hand. Wood chose the treacherous route to avoid the three USN cruisers patrolling the roadstead off the harbor, near the three-mile bell, waiting to send *Tallahassee* to a watery grave.

Fleming, pacing the *Tallahassee*'s bridge, ordered absolute silence so that he could listen to the cues of pounding surf on the rocky beaches along both sides of the narrow passage. He issued whispered, rapid-fire course changes to Commander Wood's nervous helmsman as the twin-screwed cruiser plied her way through the inky blackness. Finally Fleming heard the sound he had been waiting for—his neighbor's noisy spaniel barking on the shore, the sound that told the experienced pilot the ship had cleared the last dangerous ledge. Safe, open water now lay before the Confederate cruiser. Those on the bridge of *Tallahassee* watched in the far distance the winking navigational lights of the US Navy vessels patrolling off the main harbor entrance. Wood thanked Fleming for his help before the pilot left *Tallahassee* to row his small skiff ashore; then Wood ordered a final course change to head the darkened vessel safely out to sea, well clear of his Northern enemy.

POSTSCRIPT

Tallahassee went on to further adventures, successfully raiding and sinking numerous US vessels until she was finally seized near the end of the war by British authorities at the port of Liverpool, England. She was later turned over to the US government.

After the war John Taylor Wood escaped to Cuba, but he later returned to Halifax, became a citizen, and started a successful shipping business. His son Charles graduated from Canada's Royal Military College and was the first Canadian officer to die during the Boer War in South Africa. John Taylor Wood's grandson became a notable commissioner of the Royal Canadian Mounted Police.

Turtle *Snaps at* Eagle's *Bottom*

Amerca's first submarine was designed and constructed by Yale graduate David Bushenell (1742–1824) to sink British ships during the American Revolution.

Turtle, having a hull that looked very much like two large turtle shells fused together, was seven feet deep, almost six feet wide, and designed to be propelled forward by one human power—that being a very determined submariner cranking the strange craft's propeller. Actually two hand-cranked propellers were employed, one for propelling the vessel ahead or astern and a second for diving or surfacing in conjunction with a foot-operated ballasting system. Steering was accomplished by a tiller-rudder combination (presumably the tiller was held in the very busy operator's teeth).

In dead calm with the captain/navigator/galley slave frantically cranking and pumping, *Turtle* could attain a speed of three knots and dive to twenty feet for up to half an hour before the operator was forced to surface to avoid suffocation. Armament consisted of 150 pounds of musket powder in a mine-like package, which was to be attached by an auger to the enemy's hull, below the waterline. The powder had an ingenious clockwork timer-fuse designed to ignite the powder after the operator had cranked his way to safer waters.

In 1776 Bushenell enlisted Ezra Lee, a sergeant in Washington's Continental army, to pilot his unusual craft. Lee must have been possessed of great patriotic zeal to be willing to navigate Bushenell's little seagoing coffin in attacking British naval vessels, or at least was a man who liked living on the edge. Whatever his motivation, Lee had to have been a fine physical specimen possessed of the tremendous stamina, courage, and motor skills required to control the complicated little submersible.

The first target chosen was British Admiral Richard Howe's flagship, HMS *Eagle*, then moored in New York Harbor. With great physical effort, Lee maneuvered *Turtle* out to and under Howe's vessel, but he failed to attach the explosive mine to the enemy ship because, unknown to the Americans, *Eagle*'s bottom had been covered with experimental anti-fouling copper plates designed to slow marine growth and prevent marine borers from penetrating the wooden hull of the vessel. Evidently the copper cladding was just as effective against human borers, because it prevented Lee from being able to twist the mine's auger attachment into *Eagle*'s hull. Though unsuccessful in his attempt to destroy *Eagle*, Lee did manage to get away to safety without incident.

Unfortunately for the American cause, two additional attempts at mining enemy vessels also failed, causing Bushenell to abandon further work on the project. Eventually David Bushenell changed his name and moved to Virginia, where he set up a medical practice.

64

The Silver Plate Affair

I t's April 24, 1778. Aboard the US Sloop-of-war *Ranger*, crossing Solway Firth near the Scottish–English border, the forenoon watch has just begun. Only hours before, *Ranger*'s diminutive commander John Paul Jones ended a raid on the English port town of Whitehaven—having successfully delivered a taste of the American Revolution to King George III's back doorstep.

Jones, a rising star in America's young Continental navy, is proceeding to the southwest coast of Scotland where he intends to raid the home of Dunbar Douglas, the lord lieutenant of the stewarty of Kirkcudbright and fourth earl of Selkirk. Jones has hatched a scheme to kidnap and ransom Selkirk to secure the release of American patriots languishing in British and American jails. The earl's estate is located at St. Mary's Isle, two miles from the town of Kirkcudbright near the mouth of the River Dee—ironically, only twenty miles as the crow flies from the humble cottage where Jones was born thirty-one years ago.

At noon, Jones lands with twelve men on the shore near the Selkirk estate. When some of the area's residents encounter *Ranger*'s raiding party, they mistake it for a press gang from a British frigate. Jones learns from them that the earl of Selkirk is away in London, but that her ladyship the countess of Selkirk and some female friends, as well as the earl's seven-year-old son, are at home. (The boy, Thomas Douglas, years later as the fifth earl of Selkirk, will transport the first settlers to lands that will eventually become Manitoba and North Dakota.)

With the planned abduction of the earl now clearly impossible, the disappointed seamen begin grumbling. They feel they should have something for their pains, and a couple suggest they should sack the Selkirk mansion. To prevent this, Jones decides on a plan to satisfy his men while ensuring Lady Selkirk's safety. He instructs the two officers in the party to proceed to the house with the men, ordering that only the officers should enter the house. They are to politely demand the family silver, accept whatever they are given, then return without searching the house.

The countess of Selkirk, though surprised, receives the intruders with a brave and noble coolness that immediately earns her the respect of the American officers standing before her. Her relief at being spared the destruction of her home induces the lady to offer Jones, through the officers, an invitation to dine with her and her guests. The officers refuse on Jones's behalf, saying he would not wish to put her ladyship to any trouble. The party leaves St. Mary's shortly after the butler hands over approximately 160 pounds of silver in the form of teapots, sugar bowls, cream pitchers, and flatware from the butler's pantry, ending what must be the most bizarre operation in US Navy history.

Captain John Paul Jones and *Ranger* continued cruising Britain's coasts after the raid on the Selkirk estate, taking HMS *Drake* near Belfast on the Irish coast before returning to the French port of Brest with their English prize and the Selkirk silver. But the American captain had evidently been so impressed with the Lady Selkirk's reported *sang froid* in handling the rebel intrusion into her home that he decided to pen an eloquent and apologetic letter to the lady, explaining his actions. The letter reads in part:

> I had but a moment to think how I might gratify them [the landing party], and at the same time do your ladyship the least injury. I charged the two officers to permit none of the seamen to enter the house, or to hurt anything about it, to accept of the plate (silverware) which was offered, and to come away without making a search, or demanding anything else. I am induced to believe that I was punctually obeyed; since I am informed that the plate which they brought away is far short of the quantity expressed in the inventory which accompanied it. I have gratified my men . . .

Incredibly, Jones also added:

> . . . and when the plate is sold I shall become the purchaser, and will gratify my own feelings by restoring it to you by such conveyance as you shall please to direct.

Jones did indeed keep his word, although the infuriated earl, for more than a decade after the event, refused to accept the silver. When Selkirk finally relented and agreed to take it back, he wrote to Jones who was then living in Paris, ending his letter with the conciliatory words:

> . . . both officers and men behaved in all respects so well that it would have done credit to the best disciplined troops.

From 1778 to 1780 Captain John Paul Jones's cruising exploits in United Kingdom waters struck terror into coastal-dwelling Britishers' hearts—with the possible exception of that undaunted organ beating within the breast of the countess of Selkirk, who had witnessed a charming gallantry in the actions of *Ranger*'s captain.

One is tempted to wonder if the returned silver was present at the table when fabled Scottish poet Robert Burns, visiting the Selkirks at St. Mary's Isle in 1793, uttered his now famous "Selkirk Grace" before dinner:

> *Some ha'e meat that canna' eat,*
> *And some would eat that want it,*
> *But we ha'e meat, and we can eat,*
> *And sae the Lord be thankit.*

About the Author

Greg began working as a freelance journalist-photographer in 1995, specializing in marine subjects, especially nautical history. His writing has been published at the *Writer's Digest* Web site and in a variety of US consumer publications, including *American Yacht Review*, *Threads* magazine, *Outdoor Photographer*, *The Artilleryman* magazine, *Professional Mariner*, *Ocean Voyager*, as well as *Cruising Helmsman* magazine (Sydney, Australia), where he wrote "Tell Tales," a regular monthly column.

Greg has also written a regular marine history column for *Ocean Navigator* magazine, where his often irreverent style proved popular with readers of "Looking Astern." In addition to this column, Greg contributed technical articles on traditional celestial navigation, book and film reviews, correspondence, and photography to *Ocean Navigator*.

Greg's photography has been published in travel books produced by Reader's Digest and Windsor Publications (California), and his images have appeared in Parks Canada advertising.

Although new to fiction writing, Greg has produced a collection of short stories and completed a novel, *Inheriting Valhalla*, about the adventures of a young and fiercely independent Texas girl who inherits an old sea captain's estate in the sleepy Maine town of Searsport. At present he is writing another novel, *Stand Out to Sea*, a rollicking eighteenth-century sea yarn written in the style of Patrick O'Brian. He is also working on a stage play, a comedy in three acts titled *The Mother Factor*.

Greg lives in Dartmouth, Nova Scotia, with his wife, Donna, and an endlessly increasing collection of antique nautical books.